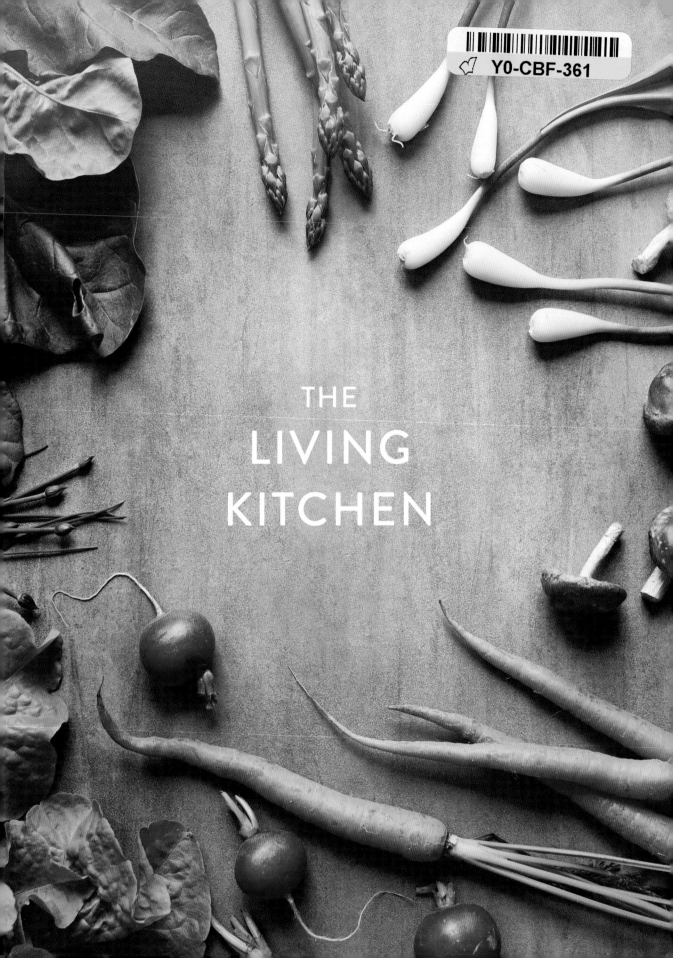

THE
LIVING
KITCHEN

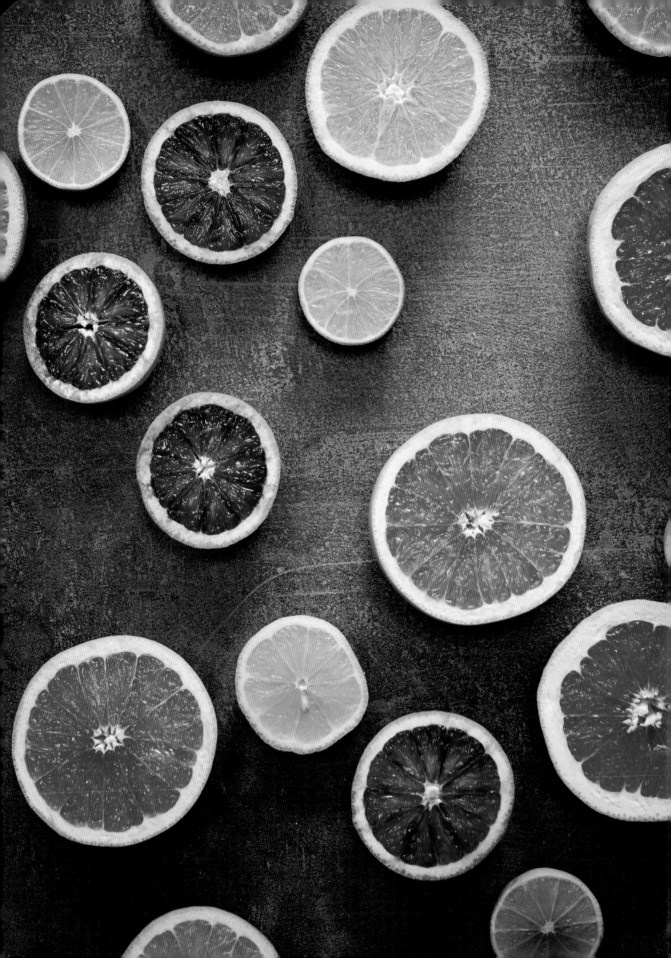

THE LIVING KITCHEN

NOURISHING WHOLE-FOOD RECIPES FOR CANCER TREATMENT AND RECOVERY

TAMARA GREEN and SARAH GROSSMAN

Photography by Daniel Alexander

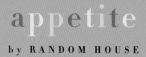

appetite
by RANDOM HOUSE

Appetite by Random House® and colophon are registered trademarks
of Penguin Random House LLC.

This publication contains the opinions and ideas of its authors. It is intended to provide
helpful and informative material on the subjects addressed in the publication. It is sold with
the understanding that the author and publisher are not engaged in rendering medical,
health, or any kind of personal professional services. Nutritional and other needs vary
depending on age, sex, and health status. If you suspect that you have a serious medical
problem, the authors strongly urge you to consult your medical, health, or other competent
professional for treatment.

Library and Archives Canada Cataloguing in Publication is available upon request.
ISBN: 9780525611479
eBook ISBN: 9780147530646

Cover design: Talia Abramson
Interior design: Kelly Hill
Cover photography: Daniel Alexander
Photographs: All Daniel Alexander except pages 3, 7, 262, which are by Jenn and Dave Stark
Food styling: Daniel Alexander, Sarah Grossman and Tamara Green

Printed and bound in China
Published in Canada by Appetite by Random House®,
a division of Penguin Random House Canada Limited.

www.penguinrandomhouse.ca

10   9   8   7   6   5   4   3   2   1

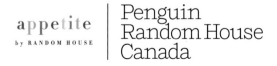

appetite
by RANDOM HOUSE

Penguin
Random House
Canada

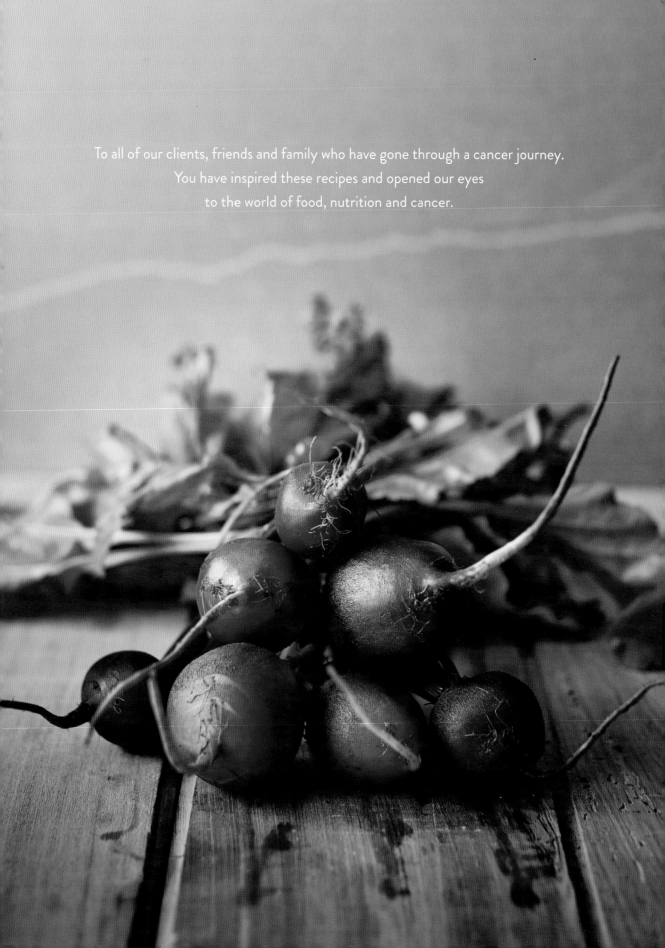

To all of our clients, friends and family who have gone through a cancer journey.
You have inspired these recipes and opened our eyes
to the world of food, nutrition and cancer.

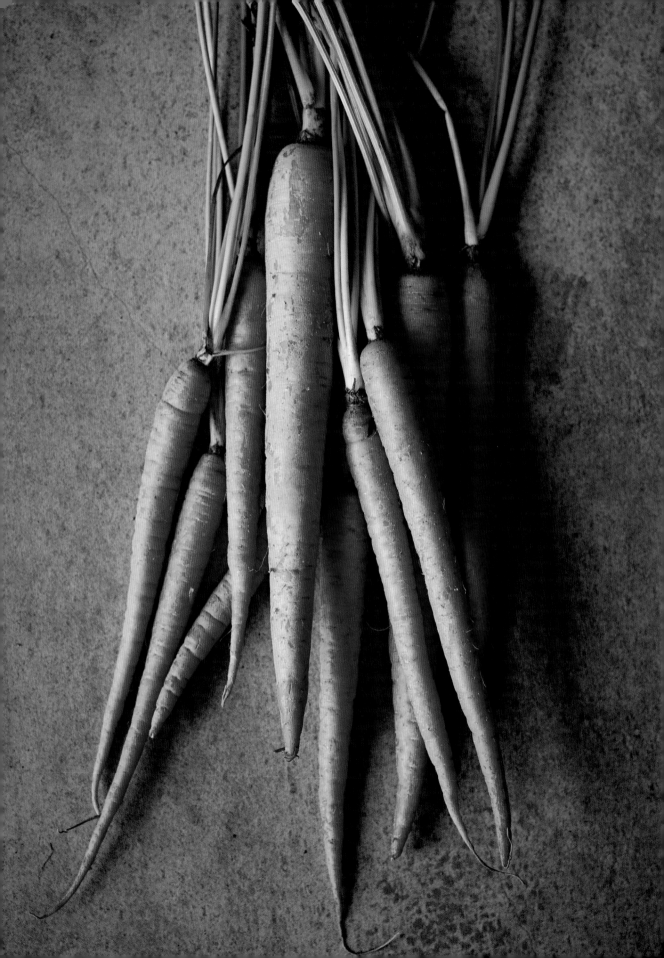

Contents

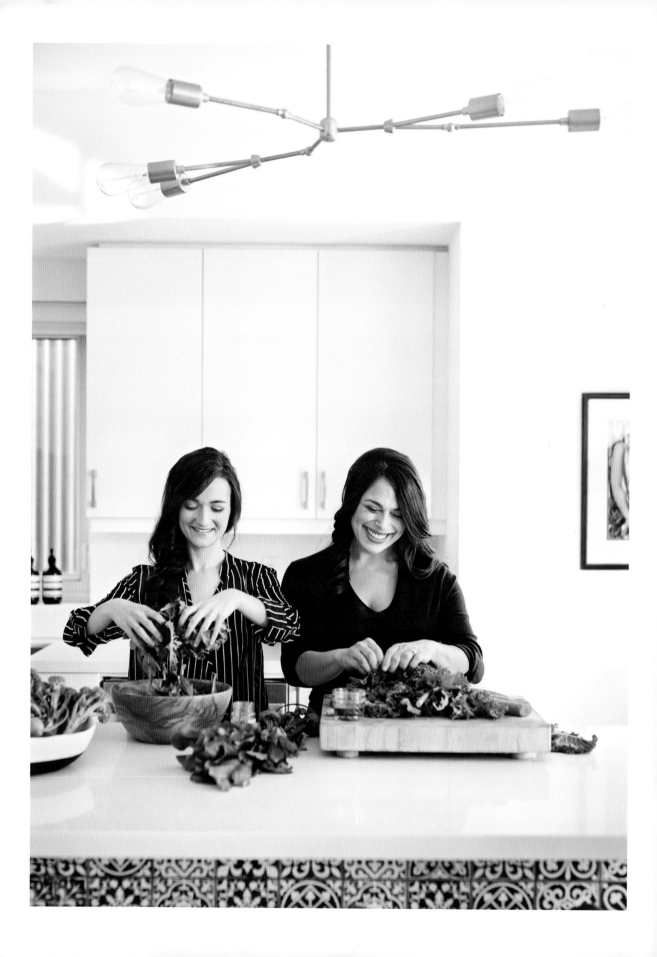

Introduction

We are honored that you picked up this book, and we are ready to share our valuable nutrition knowledge and recipes with you. It is our hope and goal that we make a real impact and difference in the lives of everyone who finds this book.

After years of working with clients as holistic nutritionists, we've been able to see firsthand how cancer has unfortunately become ever more present in the world today. Like so many of you, in recent years, we have seen very important and dear people in our lives be diagnosed with the disease. While this is frightening, there is so much we can do to help and support one another through this challenge. We know how meaningful a single action can be, whether it's preparing a meal for a friend with cancer or giving a loved one the knowledge and recipes to make their own nutritious food. And thanks to the work we do, we have seen how powerful healthy food is in supporting the body through cancer treatment. This motivates and inspires us to keep doing the work that we do, and to continue to raise awareness about cancer and the power of nutrition.

In a changing world where there is more industrialization, toxins in the environment, and unhealthy processed foods, it is more important than ever to return to whole foods and prepare meals from real ingredients. Real food is an essential part of any cancer treatment plan. After years of working with food and nutrition, and preparing more meals than we can count, we have put our knowledge into our first cookbook—which you're reading now!

Our story together began at the Institute of Holistic Nutrition in Toronto in 2009, where we met and immediately bonded over our shared love of good, wholesome food. We launched our company, Living Kitchen, in 2010 and since then have offered nutrition counseling, cooking instruction, meal delivery, and private chef cooking services. We prepare food for clients and develop recipes to meet the dietary needs of various health conditions, like irritable bowel syndrome, inflammatory bowel disease, colitis, ulcers, Crohn's disease, fibromyalgia, multiple sclerosis, hormonal imbalances, diabetes, depression, infertility, obesity, chronic fatigue syndrome, and weakened immune systems. We cook to accommodate food allergies and to make meals that support recovery from illness. We've seen firsthand the impact that nutritious food has on helping our clients manage all of these conditions and improving their physical, mental, and emotional health. For this reason, food has always been at the core of our work.

Cancer support and prevention became a primary focus of our work in the spring of 2012. Both of us had lost family members to cancer in the past, but at that point young friends of ours were diagnosed, which, until then, had been unheard-of to us. As more friends and family members were being diagnosed with this disease, we felt strongly called to work with cancer patients. So with passion, purpose, and knowledge, we began working hard to nutritionally support people undergoing cancer treatment—to strengthen their bodies to help them recover. Since then we have worked intimately with people touched by cancer, learning about their experiences and developing meal plans and specialized recipes to help them through their treatment and recovery.

Sharing our knowledge feels vital to us; it is truly the most important thing we can do. We're ready for our cookbook to empower readers to learn, cook, and recover.

With health,
Sarah + Tamara

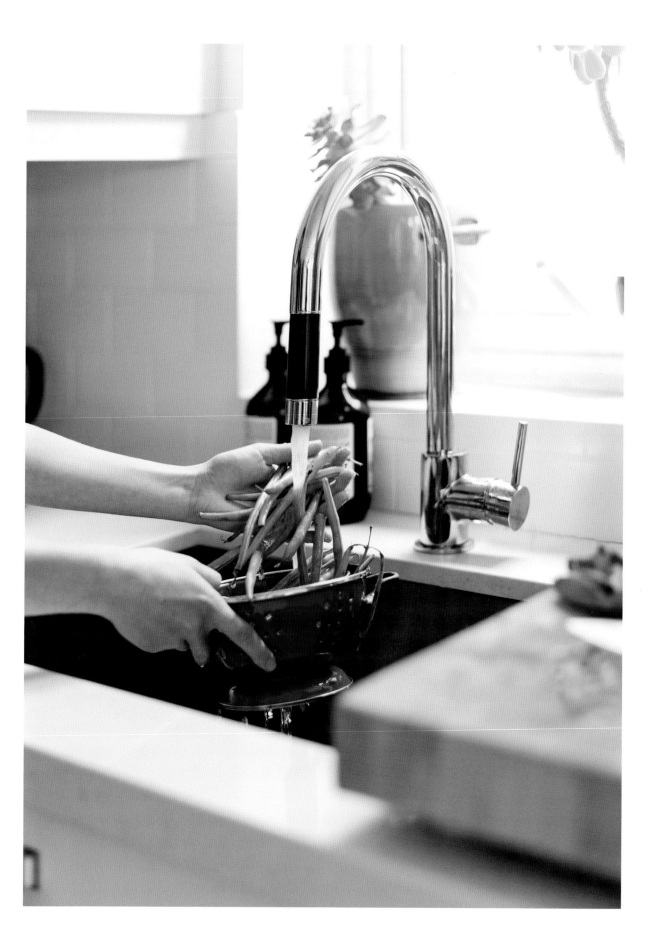

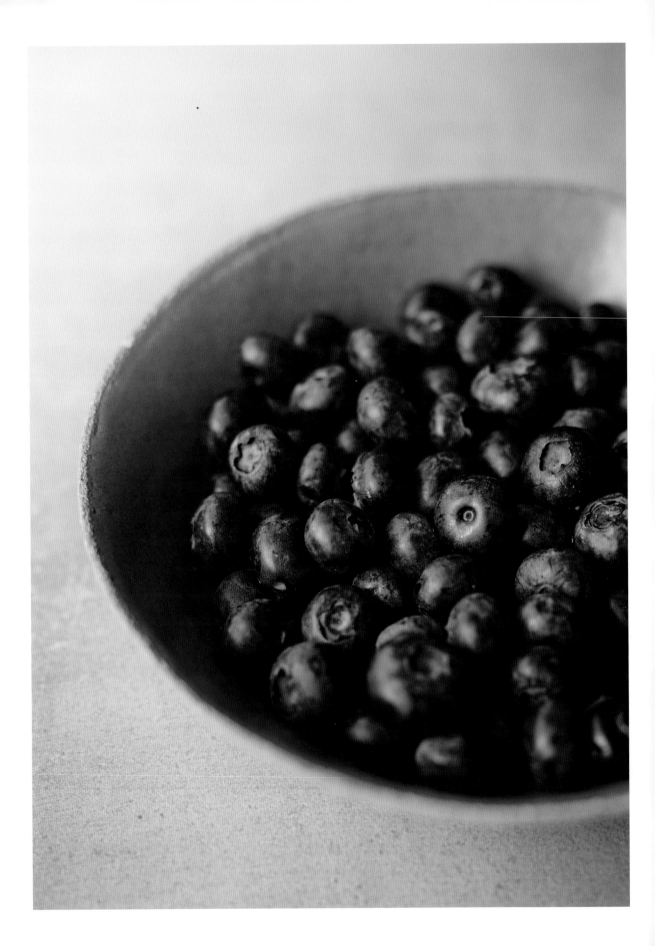

CHAPTER ONE

Facing a Diagnosis

Welcome to your new cancer food guide. Whomever and wherever you are in the cancer journey—whether you're a loving bystander helping a family member or a friend, or you've recently been diagnosed, or you're receiving treatment, or you're in remission—we're writing this for you. We're your guiding hands to walk you through this, bite by bite. Follow along as we explore important nutrition information and recipes that will support you before, during, and after treatment.

There is undoubtedly a lot changing in your life right now as you process what is happening. What you eat, how you eat, and your relationship with food is about to change—your appetite may decrease, you may lose your sense of taste, or you may be nauseated to eat. We promise to guide you through this process. Before we dive into the recipes, we want to give you a little background on the fundamentals of nutrition, how to eat when you experience side effects, and how to prep your kitchen to set you up for success. Let's get started.

PROPER NUTRITION IS KEY

Hearing the words "You have cancer" is an overwhelming and scary experience. During this time, you and your loved ones will work closely with your health care team to figure out the best plan for you. Regardless of the treatment, be it surgery, chemotherapy, radiation, or alternative theraphies, supporting your body through your diet is essential. Proper nutrition can help keep your body strong as it undergoes intense therapies to kill cancer cells, and what you eat can mitigate common side effects like nausea, loss of appetite, and fatigue. Colorful vegetables and fruits, healthy proteins, and good fats possess antitumor, antiangiogenesis,* antioxidant, anti-inflammatory, and antimutagenic properties. This means that many of the foods you can eat have powerful anticancer nutrients that work to support your health and recovery. These foods act synergistically with each other and with treatments to help speed up recovery time and make some therapies more effective.

SAFE, SUPPORTIVE, AND NOURISHING RECIPES

The recipes in this book are designed to be easy to prepare, wholesome, and delicious. They are meant to be enjoyed by you, your loved ones, and caregivers. We have created this book to feed everyone. What you eat right now, following your diagnosis or during treatment, is important for your health and recovery. But we believe that eating should not be an added stress on top of everything else you're going through, so we want to make it as simple and as tasty as possible. Our recipes work with all types of treatments and are intended to lessen side effects, as well as guide you on what to eat before, during and after cancer.

Medical treatments can be effective at killing cancer cells; however, they also harm normal cells in the process. This harm is what leads to side effects (hair loss, nausea, vomiting, constipation, diarrhea, dry mouth, taste changes, suppressed immunity, low white and red blood cell counts, and fatigue) in the areas of the body where there is constant and normal cell division, growth, and repair, like the digestive tract, mouth, hair, skin, and bone marrow. Please remember that everyone experiences symptoms differently and at different stages during treatment, so what happens to one person may not happen to you.

WHAT DO I EAT NOW?

The big question we get asked by our clients is "What do I eat now?" There is a lot of concern before and during treatment about what to eat, and many people are also concerned about what their families will eat while they're off receiving treatment. We always encourage our clients to eat a plant-based diet that includes whole, unrefined foods made from scratch. And while we've seen different diets (such as vegetarian, ketogenic, and

---

* Angiogenesis is the formation of new blood vessels—a process that tumors need in order to grow and spread.

gluten-free) work for different people, as nutritionists, we don't feel there's one "best" diet. But we do know one thing: The common thread between all these different diets is the importance of eating an abundance of fresh produce. You'll learn much more about what to eat during treatment in Chapter 2.

WHAT YOU EAT INFLUENCES YOUR GENETICS

Epigenetics is the study of how your genes express themselves without actually changing your underlying DNA. Though it's been around since the 1940s, scientists began making breakthroughs in research in the 2000s, and continue to. Epigenetics is incredibly exciting for cancer research, and here's why: there is growing research showing that certain nutrients found in many foods, such as turmeric, broccoli, kale, cauliflower, grapes, garlic, soy, onions, fish oil, and green tea can turn your genes off and on to reverse abnormal gene activations. Your genetic code doesn't change, but the way your genes express themselves does. Think about it this way: your diet may have the power to actually reprogram your health, *despite* your genetics.

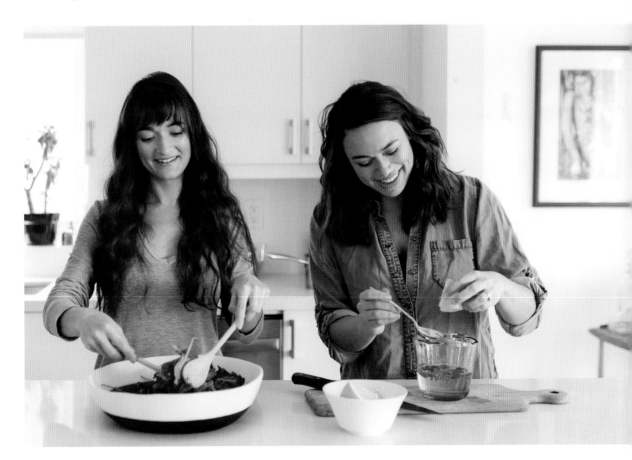

We've made sure to include the foods mentioned above and other power-house ingredients (check out our comprehensive list in chapter 2) in our recipes. Eating them together and as whole foods rather than as isolated supplemental nutrients provides a greater and safer benefit.

YOUR APPETITE WILL CHANGE

Eating during treatment may not be easy. Your appetite or tastes may change, you may experience dry mouth or sores, or you may have no energy to cook. We get it. So we've developed specific recipes designed for you during these stages. Our soups, smoothies, juices, elixirs, sauces, marinades, and dressings will be essential during this time, providing your body with nutrients in a noninvasive, gentle way. When your appetite is strong, and substantial foods are appealing to you, this is the time to eat and eat well, so use our recipes for main dishes, snacks, and sides and make them a part of your treatment plan.

RELEASING FOOD FEAR WITH FOOD MINDFULNESS

When you or someone close to you has cancer, there may be a lot of fear that surrounds eating. Whether you're anxious before a treatment, nervous that you'll experience side effects, or just unsure what to eat, it can all weigh very heavily on you. It can feel disempowering to lack control over your diet and health, so this is where we encourage our clients to bring food mindfulness into play. This concept promotes the idea that it's not just about *what* you eat, but *how* you eat and the thoughts you have around your diet. Your body actually digests and absorbs nutrients better when it is in a relaxed state. This state is known as "rest and digest," and it's when your body's parasympathetic nervous system is stimulated.

If you're having trouble eating, if you can, before you are about to eat, focus on getting into a state of relaxation. Everyone has their own way of achieving this, but we find deep breathing, visualizations, and affirmations work remarkably well. Your mind is incredibly powerful and can actually change the way your body responds to the food you eat and how you feel. Become aware of the thoughts and language you use around the foods you eat or don't eat and the positive or negative labels you attribute to your food and eating habits. This language can impact the food you eat and your appetite. See the box for our guide to getting into a relaxed state.

Breathing Exercise before Eating

Before sitting down to a meal, begin a one- to five-minute breathing exercise (it can be longer too, if you want). All this requires is taking deep breaths in through your nose and out through your mouth, imagining that you're sending the breaths all the way down to your belly. Simple, right? If you want, you can add a visualization—simply close your eyes and picture yourself in a peaceful place, calmly eating.

You can also include an affirmation with each breath. Choose something that feels right for you. Here are some examples:

"I eat with ease and peace; my body absorbs and uses the nutrients it needs."

"This meal is full of the exact nutrients I need."

"I release fear and allow my body to take in what it needs."

"My body knows exactly what to do and easily digests everything I eat."

Even if whatever affirmation you choose feels untrue to you, saying it tells your body that this is what it needs to do. You don't even need to say the affirmation out loud; you can simply repeat the affirmation in your mind.

Maybe food mindfulness sounds a little out there for you, but it truly is an important part of eating for every person. When you lack control, especially with respect to your health, food mindfulness is one area that may bring you power, so if eating becomes very challenging for you, we recommend introducing this practice. The results may surprise you.

HOW TO USE THIS BOOK

The first thing to know about this book is that you can't get it wrong. There is no wrong way to use this book. Our chapters are laid out deliberately to help build up your nutrition knowledge, to show you techniques to combat side effects and guide you on how to buy the "right" ingredients, but if you feel like one particular chapter calls to you more than the others, feel free to start there. If you feel inclined to follow the book as we've organized it, we highly recommend reading chapters 2 and 3 next. These chapters introduce you to the fundamentals of nutrition and show you which foods are important to add to your diet right now and which foods to remove immediately. We've noticed that when our clients learn foundational nutrition concepts and understand *why* significant dietary changes are important, they are more likely to transform their diet and eat to support their health and recovery, even when it's challenging.

Each recipe is equipped with icons that inform you which side effects it aims to help. To stimulate your appetite, carefully flip through the photographs and see which recipes look most appealing. We begin our digestive process with our eyes first, so the photos can actually help get your appetite going.

If you don't have the energy to cook for yourself at the moment, try to find someone in your life who will, or hire a company like ours to cook for you. During the cancer process, the people around you often want to help but just don't know how. Cooking for you is a truly meaningful way for them to support you. If you don't have anyone in your life who can cook, that's OK too. Many of our recipes can actually be made ahead and frozen, so cook when you have energy, freeze, and simply defrost and heat when you're not feeling up to cooking.

Here's a quick breakdown of the chapters so you know what's ahead.

CHAPTER 2: "LET FOOD BE THY MEDICINE"
This chapter is a minicourse in Nutrition 101. It covers the basic nutrition principles, explaining what fats, carbohydrates, proteins, vitamins, and minerals are and how to include them in your diet. We also break down popular nutrition lingo like "omega-3," "antioxidant," and "phytonutrient."

CHAPTER 3: FUNCTIONAL AND DYSFUNCTIONAL FOODS
Here, we provide a comprehensive list of functional foods that we recommend including in your diet during treatment. We also outline dysfunctional foods to eliminate, because they contribute to illness and provide minimal to no health benefits.

CHAPTER 4: EATING TO COMBAT COMMON SIDE EFFECTS

Chapter 4 may be the most important chapter for you. This is where we explain specifically how to mitigate side effects and we provide you with guiding menu plans, which are one of the most helpful tools in this book. This chapter gives you that important information about what to eat before, during, and after treatment.

CHAPTER 5: PREPARING THE KITCHEN

Before making big dietary changes, it's always a good idea to clean house and get your kitchen in order. This means purging unhealthy cookware and ingredients. We go over how to buy organic food on a budget and what to look out for when buying different ingredients.

THE RECIPES

The recipes are the heart of this cookbook. This section is where you take everything you've learned in the previous chapters and put it into physical practice. Knowing this information is only half of it; eating is the next step, and our recipes will help bring the information to life. As mentioned earlier, each recipe is equipped with icons that will let you know which symptoms it's helpful for.

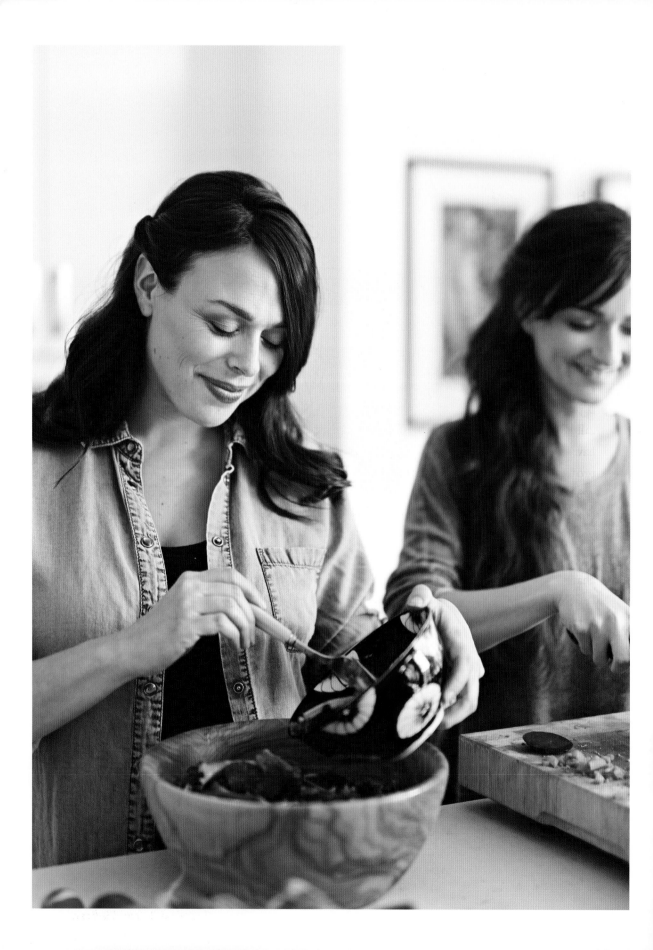

CHAPTER TWO

"Let Food Be Thy Medicine"

A Minicourse in Nutrition

"Let food be thy medicine and medicine be thy food" —HIPPOCRATES

As holistic nutritionists we believe that diet and nutrition can be used as an adjunct therapy during cancer treatment to strengthen, restore, and physically heal the body. The nutritious, unprocessed, whole foods that you eat have powerful enzymes, minerals, vitamins, antioxidants, phytonutrients, proteins, fats, and carbohydrates that all work together to support the body, stimulate the immune system, regulate cell cycles, strengthen the muscles, build the bones, cushion and support the organs, detoxify the blood, stabilize the blood sugar, and much, much more.

Depending on your diagnosis and course of treatment, your diet may change from the way it's been. You may develop aversions to foods you once loved, you may have a new desire to eat as cleanly as possible, or you may be unable to eat food with certain textures and tastes. Our recipes and meal plans work with you, so that no matter how your diet evolves, you will be nourished.

But before we get specific about what to eat, we're going to take it back to the nutrition basics and break down how the foods you eat affect your overall health and body.

THE MACRONUTRIENTS

Macronutrients—fat, carbohydrates, and protein—are the major food components that your body needs to function. In this section, we'll explain what they are and what they do for you.

Fat insulates the body, controls internal temperature, and keeps you warm. You need it to absorb and transport key nutrients like vitamins A, D, E, and K, all of which have unique responsibilities such as supporting the immune system and reversing damage that could lead to cancer. Fats are an important component of cell membranes, which protect the cells' internal DNA from mutations, damage, and infection. They provide the body with energy and protect vital organs, including the heart and the brain. They also build hormones and help cells communicate with each other. Clearly, fats have a lot of work to do.

There are many types of fats out there, like saturated fat (found in coconut oil, beef, and poultry), monounsaturated fat (extra-virgin olive oil has it), and polyunsaturated fat (found in nuts, seeds, and fish). You need them all.

ARE YOU READY TO GET A BIT SCIENCE-Y?

You may have heard about the two types of essential fatty acids, omega-3 and omega-6. These have a variety of functions in the body, but the most important thing they do is make prostaglandins, which are hormone-like substances that regulate inflammation in the body.

Omega-6 fatty acids make two types of prostaglandins: The first is responsible for preventing blood clots and other beneficial processes. The second type does the opposite: it promotes tumor cell proliferation, cancer progression, blood clotting, and inflammation, and it suppresses immune function.

Omega-3 fatty acids make the third type of prostaglandin, which reduces inflammation in the body and defends against infections. Studies show these prostaglandins kill cancer cells, prevent metastasis (when cancer spreads from one area to other locations in the body), and enhance the effectiveness of anticancer treatments, while possibly reducing their side effects like weight loss. They're basically nutrition superheroes.

Everyone needs both omega-6 and omega-3 fatty acids in their diet. However, Western diets are much higher in omega-6 fats (found in processed foods and vegetable oils) than omega-3 fatty acids (which you'll find in nuts, seeds, and cold-water fish), because the dietary sources of omega-3 fatty acids are not eaten as frequently as the foods that contain omega-6 fatty acids. This contributes to chronic underlying inflammation in the body.

WHAT FATS SHOULD YOU EAT?

These are our favorite fats for you to eat as you prepare for, go through, and recover from treatment.

PLANT-BASED FATS

Sources: Nuts* and seeds, coconut products, avocados, and olives.

ANIMAL FATS

Sources: Organic, pasture-raised, or hormone- and antibiotic-free chicken and turkey; organic, pasture-raised or free-range eggs; wild, sustainably caught, or sustainably farmed fish; and pasture-raised lamb and beef.

OMEGA-3-RICH FOODS

Sources: Flax oil and seeds; hemp oil and seeds; chia seeds; sesame seeds and oil; walnuts; cold-water fish like salmon, halibut, cod, trout, mackerel, and sardines.

OILS

There are so many different oils out there, and it's important to choose the right one for what you're eating and cooking. Some oils are very sensitive to heat, light, and air. These should only be heated to a specific temperature or not used for cooking at all, because when sensitive oils are heated beyond their smoke point, they break down and become toxic. There are other oils that won't be damaged from high-heat cooking. Be sure to buy oils in dark glass bottles, rather than clear plastic ones, as this will protect them from oxidation.

---

* Peanuts can contain a carcinogenic toxin called "aflatoxin," which has been linked to liver cancer, so we recommend limiting your consumption of them.

TYPE OF OIL	SAFE TEMP (MAX. HEAT)	WHY WE LIKE IT	WHY WE DON'T LIKE IT	WHEN TO USE IT
Extra-Virgin Olive Oil (EVOO)	350°F–410°F	Extra-virgin olive oil is unrefined and it protects cells' genetic material from damage. It has anti-inflammatory and antioxidant properties. A good-quality, expensive EVOO can be heated to 410°F. If you know you're not using the best quality, don't heat it beyond 375°F. When purchasing, ensure the label says "extra-virgin olive oil," otherwise it is a refined version.		Use it to lightly sauté, bake, or roast at medium temperatures; use it in salad dressings and marinades, and to drizzle over raw and cooked vegetables or veg-etarian or animal proteins.
Virgin, Unrefined Coconut Oil	350°F	Coconut oil holds up well to medium-high temperatures, making it excellent for cooking. It's easy to digest. Studies conducted with tra-ditionally prepared coconut oil have shown that it lowers cholesterol, while refined coconut oil has been shown to raise cholesterol. When purchasing, ensure the label says "unrefined" or "virgin," otherwise it is a refined version.		Use it to sauté, bake, or roast vegetables and vege-tarian or animal proteins at medium temperatures. Use it in baked goods, where it can replace butter or oils. Put it in smoothies or spread it over breakfast items like healthy muffins, toast, or pancakes.
Flax Oil and Hemp Oil	Do not heat. Store in the refrigerator.	Flax and hemp oil are rich in omega-3 fatty acids and have anti-inflammatory benefits.		Use it in salad dressings and smoothies. Drizzle over cooked or raw vegetables, or over yogurt, cereal, chia pudding, or healthy pancakes. Never heat these oils.
Unrefined Toasted Sesame Oil	350°F	Toasted sesame oil is best for dressings, marinades, and light sautéing because of its strong, nutty flavor.		Use it in salad dressings, sauces, and marinades, and as a flavor enhancer.

TYPE OF OIL	SAFE TEMP (MAX. HEAT)	WHY WE LIKE IT	WHY WE DON'T LIKE IT	WHEN TO USE IT
Butter	350°F	Butter contains healthy saturated fats that stand up to higher temperatures, not to mention it tastes delicious. The fat in butter feeds good bacteria in the gut and is easy to digest. Always choose butter over margarine.		Use it to sauté, bake, or roast vegetables and vegetarian or animal proteins. Use it in baked goods or spread it over healthy muffins, toast, or pancakes. We recommend buying organic or grass-fed butter.
Ghee (Clarified Butter)	350°F	Ghee is traditionally used as a healing oil in Ayurvedic medicine. It's made from butter, but doesn't contain lactose or casein, as the milk solids have been removed. It benefits the digestive tract. Studies have found that ghee is linked with reduced growth of cancer, specifically in mammary glands.		Use it to sauté or roast vegetables and vegetarian or animal proteins. Use it in baked goods or spread it over healthy muffins, toast, or pancakes. We recommend buying organic ghee.
Refined Avocado Oil	520°F		Despite it being refined, which removes many of the health benefits, we sometimes recommend avocado oil for high-heat cooking. (Note that some companies are conscious of the refining process and do not use harsh chemicals to extract the oil.)	Use it in moderation. Use it to sauté, bake, or roast vegetables and vegetarian or animal proteins, if you're doing so at very high temperatures.
Vegetable Oils: Refined Canola, Safflower, Sunflower, and Soybean	400°F–450°F		Vegetable oils have gone through a refining process that has destroyed their valuable nutritional properties.	We recommend you don't use these oils.

CARBS ARE YOUR MAIN FUEL SOURCE:
HERE'S WHAT YOU NEED TO KNOW

You need carbs to supply energy, eliminate waste, and support a healthy immune system, nervous system, and muscle function. There are two major classifications of carbohydrates: simple sugars and complex carbohydrates.

SIMPLE SUGARS AND REFINED CARBOHYDRATES:
THE SUGARS YOU CRAVE

Simple sugars, also known as simple carbohydrates, aren't complex structures, like their older, wiser cousins the complex carb (more on them below). Simple sugars break down in the body very quickly. They're found in fruit; all sweeteners, including white sugar, brown sugar, and natural sweeteners like maple syrup and honey; and candy. Another type of simple carbohydrate is highly refined carbohydrates. These are found in white flour, white rice, and white pasta. Many baked goods combine white flour with lots of sweeteners for a double dose.

All carbohydrates break down into glucose, the main simple sugar used by tissues and cells for energy, but the problem with simple carbohydrates is the speed at which they are digested and the amount that people consume. Eating too many simple and refined sugars stresses out the pancreas and leads to nutrient deficiencies in the body. During cancer treatment, you need your body to function to the best of its ability to rebuild healthy cells and maintain strength. It's really important to reduce your intake of simple sugars—even natural ones like pure maple syrup—and most importantly refined carbohydrates.

COMPLEX CARBS: IT'S NOT THAT COMPLEX, WE PROMISE

Complex carbohydrates are structurally complex, so it takes the body longer to break them down. This in turn prevents blood sugar spikes, which is why these carbs are often referred to as "low glycemic." Good sources of complex carbs are lower in sugar and higher in fiber, protein, and fat, all of which slows their effect on blood sugar. Examples of good complex carb sources include starchy vegetables, green vegetables, some types of fruit, whole grains, nuts, seeds, legumes, and beans.

FIBER: YOUR GUT'S BEST FRIEND

The gut is the seat of the body's immune system because of the billions of microflora that live there, protecting the body against foreign viruses, bacteria, and toxins and helping digest food. Fiber feeds these microflora, helping them grow and protect the colon. Fiber is also essential for removing toxins and waste from the intestinal tract. You can find fiber in pretty much all plant foods—vegetables, fruit, grains, legumes, beans, nuts, seeds—but remember that it is processed out of whole grains and whole rice to make refined versions like white flour and white rice.

BURNING QUESTION: DOES SUGAR FEED CANCER?

The relationship between sugar and cancer is continuously being researched and studied. All cells in the body use glucose (sugar) for energy, including cancerous cells. In 1924, Otto Warburg observed that cancer cells metabolize glucose differently from normal cells. From Warburg's findings many people theorized that refined sugar feeds cancer, and the way to starve cancer is to cut off its food supply: that is, stop eating sugar. But, it isn't just refined sugar that eventually breaks down into glucose in the body; simple sugars and complex carbs, like blueberries, brown rice, and sweet potatoes do too. So what ends up being more important is the *quality* and *type* of carbohydrate being consumed. Some people opt for a ketogenic diet during treatment because this diet eliminates almost all carbohydrates so your body burns fat rather than glucose.

Refined grains and sugars are essentially empty calories. They provide the body with minimal to no nutrition, and they lead to elevated blood sugar and insulin levels that promote fat storage and inflammation, and in turn heighten cancer risk. This is why it's ideal to eat more unrefined complex carbohydrates instead of refined ones. Insulin increases other hormones known as insulin-like growth factors. This can enhance tumor growth and is known to increase the risk of breast, prostate, colon, and lung cancers.

The takeaway here, from our perspective, is to cut out or limit refined grains and sugars from your diet and focus on eating high-quality carbs like whole grains, legumes, beans, and colorful vegetables.

IS GOING GLUTEN-FREE RIGHT FOR YOU?

Gluten is a protein found in the grains spelt, rye, kamut, and barley, but it's most abundant in wheat. It's the sticky substance that makes baked goods and bread fluffy, airy, light, and elastic and helps them rise. In the gut, though, gluten can stick to the intestinal tract and, for people who suffer from celiac disease or gluten intolerance, this can cause painful side effects, including an inability to absorb nutrients and damage to the intestinal tract. Even some people who don't have an intolerance avoid or limit gluten because they feel it impacts their gut health. There is no diagnostic test to detect gluten sensitivity; however, some people have found that unwanted symptoms, like digestive discomfort, mental fog, fatigue, headaches, eczema, joint pain, and nausea, have decreased after eliminating gluten.

REMEMBER Just because something is gluten-free does not mean it is healthy. Read labels and make sure there are no refined sugars, unwanted preservatives, or refined oils lurking in the gluten-free products you buy.

As nutritionists, we believe "every body" is different and therefore everyone tolerates gluten differently—so it's important that you decide for yourself how gluten makes you feel. If your digestive system feels compromised during cancer treatment, then eliminating or limiting gluten, or more so wheat, may be beneficial for you. If you have an underlying sensitivity that may be compromising your digestion, it's important that it doesn't interfere with your health right now. But, if eliminating gluten feels too extreme, simply limit it or choose alternative grains like spelt, kamut, and rye.

PROTEIN IS IN CHARGE OF REPAIRING AND MAINTAINING YOUR BODY: HERE'S HOW

Protein helps build skin, bone, hair, eyes, nails, muscles, and tissues and regulates the activity of your internal organs, including your heart and brain. Protein is also especially essential for healing and recovery. During treatment, it helps to maintain weight, prevents muscle wasting and fatigue, and promotes tissue repair. Eating healthy sources of protein also helps regulate blood sugar, improve energy if you feel tired and fatigued, and prevent crashes in energy. Most importantly, though, when it comes to cancer treatment, protein builds antibodies that protect the body from infection. It will also help speed up recovery during treatment, especially when the body has an increased demand and need for nutrients.

WHAT PROTEIN SHOULD YOU EAT?

When your body doesn't get enough protein, it starts breaking down muscle in order to find the building blocks it needs to make it, leading to weight loss. So it's vital that you eat the right sources, especially before, during, and after treatment. Both omnivore and vegetarian or vegan sources of protein can provide the building blocks (essential amino acids) that your body needs for strength and repair.

ANIMAL PROTEINS

Animal foods like fermented dairy, eggs, poultry, meat, and fish contain all of the building blocks (essential amino acids) to build proteins.

VEGETARIAN PROTEINS

Beans, legumes, grains, nuts, seeds, and vegan protein powder all fall into this category. When you're eating non-animal, plant-based protein sources like these, it's important to eat a variety of them throughout the day, since they contain different amounts of essential amino acids, and this will ensure you get all of them.

KISS SUPPLEMENTAL NUTRITION DRINKS GOODBYE

As you're going through treatment, there's a good chance that your health-care team will recommend supplemental nutritional drinks to you. These drinks seem to have health benefits: they're a quick source of calories and protein, and they're easy to drink. Unfortunately, in our opinion as nutritionists, some of their ingredients are harmful and you should avoid them, especially when you're going through cancer care. Stick to eating whole-food sources of protein or homemade protein-rich smoothies rather than drinking processed and refined protein drinks. We have our own high-protein, easy-to-digest drinks in our smoothie chapter that actually nourish you without refined sugars, artificial sweeteners, or preservatives.

WATER, WATER, EVERYWHERE . . . BUT YOU'RE PROBABLY NOT DRINKING ENOUGH

Even though all your bodily functions rely on it, it's easy to forget how vital water is for the body. All cells need water to survive. You use it to generate energy, to transport nutrients around your body, and to eliminate toxins and waste. Each day you lose water through your skin, urine, bowels, and lungs, and you need to restore these losses by eating fruits and vegetables—and by drinking water. During treatment it's especially easy to get dehydrated from side effects such as diarrhea or vomiting, but it's also possible to become dehydrated by simply not drinking enough water, or opting for soda, black tea, or coffee instead. It's important to drink six to eight 8-ounce glasses of water a day, and you may need more depending on what side effects you're experiencing. We encourage you to try to drink water between meals instead of during them so that you don't compromise your digestion. If drinking water is a challenge, try to make it more appealing by drinking through a straw, serving the water at room temperature, or adding lemon, cucumber, or fresh mint leaves.

THE MICRONUTRIENTS: VITAMINS AND MINERALS

Micronutrients are essential nutrients that your body needs in small amounts. Like macronutrients, they are important for your health, but you eat them in much smaller quantities than carbs, fats, and proteins.

VITAMINS AND MINERALS DO ALL OF THE WORK

Your body needs vitamins for growth and tissue healing, tumor size reduction, normal cell division and growth, bone formation, protection against oxidation and free radicals, blood clotting, digestion, food metabolism, relaxation, energy, immunity stimulation, waste elimination, and disease prevention . . . so basically, everything.

It is best to get your vitamins from plant and animal sources—that is, from real food like fruits and veggies, not *just* from supplements and pills. To ensure you get a variety of vitamins in your diet, eat the rainbow, load your plate with colorful vegetables, fruit, nuts, and seeds, and lean proteins to get your vitamin fill. Some vitamins are sensitive to light, air, heat, and time, so it's important not to overcook food, as you can lose the nutrients.

Minerals come from the earth. As with vitamins, your body uses minerals to perform key daily functions and tasks in the body, like tissue and cell repair, heart function, digestion, immunity, muscle contraction and relaxation, acid-alkaline balance in the blood and tissues, and protecting cells from free radical damage. It's important to eat an array of different whole foods, like vegetables, nuts and seeds, whole grains, seafood, and eggs, to ensure that your body has access to a variety of minerals at each meal.

ANTIOXIDANTS ARE POWERFUL—HERE'S WHY

Free radicals are unpaired electrons that create damage in your body. As they try to find another electron to pair with, they create oxidative stress in the form of mutations to cells. They're mainly produced by pollution, poor diet, certain cooking methods, smoking—and chemotherapy and radiation. Antioxidants help combat oxidative stress by neutralizing and pairing with free radicals, inhibiting them from creating harm and damaging cells.

Antioxidants can be found in vitamins, minerals, phytonutrients, and amino acids. Food sources include walnuts, sunflower seeds, almonds, raw cacao, goji berries, blueberries, Brussels sprouts, broccoli, kale, cauliflower, avocados, sweet potato, carrots, onions, garlic, and green tea.

There is some controversy in the idea of taking antioxidant supplements during treatment. While some studies have found that antioxidants actually improve the effectiveness of treatment and side effects, what's safest and most important is getting antioxidants from whole food sources rather than pills, especially while undergoing treatment. Whole foods offer the body more than just antioxidants themselves; they also provide fiber, omega-3s, vitamins, and minerals.

PHYTONUTRIENTS: THE FIERCEST PLANT CHEMICALS

Phytonutrients, or phytochemicals, are plant compounds that have major protective properties and give plants their color, taste, and smell. One of the reasons we want you to "eat the rainbow" and make sure your plate is filled with colorful fruits and vegetables is so that you will get a variety of phytonutrients in your diet.

There has been a lot of research attention on phytonutrients and their association with cancer treatment and prevention. Phytonutrients have potent anticancer properties that work in unique ways to decrease abnormal cell growth, inhibit the spread of cancer cells and formation of their new blood vessels, and promote cancer cell death. Similar to antioxidants, phytonutrients are more effective when eaten together instead of separately.

There are too many phytonutrients to name, but here are a few of the major players.

PHYTONUTRIENT	FOODS YOU CAN FIND THEM IN	BENEFITS
Anthocyanins	Blackberries, blueberries, cherries, oranges, pomegranate, purple corn, raspberries	Anti-inflammatory and antioxidant.
Beta-Carotene	Carrots, leafy greens, pumpkin, squash, sweet potato	Anticarcinogenic, stimulates DNA repair enzymes, and stimulates the signal to send cells to inflammation sites.
Curcumin	Turmeric	Inhibits cancer cell growth, powerful antioxidant, anti-inflammatory, and antimutagenic.
Epigallocatechin Gallate (EGCG)	Grapes, green tea	Antioxidant, anti-inflammatory, and inhibits tumors and new blood vessels from growing.
Ferulic Acid, Caffeic Acid, Ellagic Acid	Blackberries, cabbage, cantaloupe, green tea, honeydew melon, oats, pineapple, raspberries, rice, spinach, strawberries	Induces apoptosis (cancer cell death), inhibits metastasis, and has antioxidant properties.
Genistein and Daidzein	Soy (tofu, tempeh, soybeans, miso)	Inhibits the growth of most hormone-dependent cancer cells.
Limonene	Citrus fruits, root vegetables	Promotes detoxification enzymes in the liver.
Lycopene	Apricots, papaya, pink guava, red tomatoes, watermelon	Powerful antioxidant. Slows down the formation of free radicals and can destroy them. Lowers the risk of prostate cancer.
Quercetin	Apples, broccoli, berries, buckwheat, green tea, kale, leeks, onions, red grapes	Potent antioxidant and may inhibit tumor production.
Resveratrol	Blueberries, red grapes, red wine	Inhibits proliferation of cancer cells, induces cancer cell death, delays tumor growth, reduces metastasis.
Sulforaphane and Indoles	Cruciferous vegetables (broccoli, broccoli sprouts, kale, cabbage, cauliflower), garlic, onions	Protects against cancer and mutations. Activates liver detoxification enzymes to break down carcinogens.

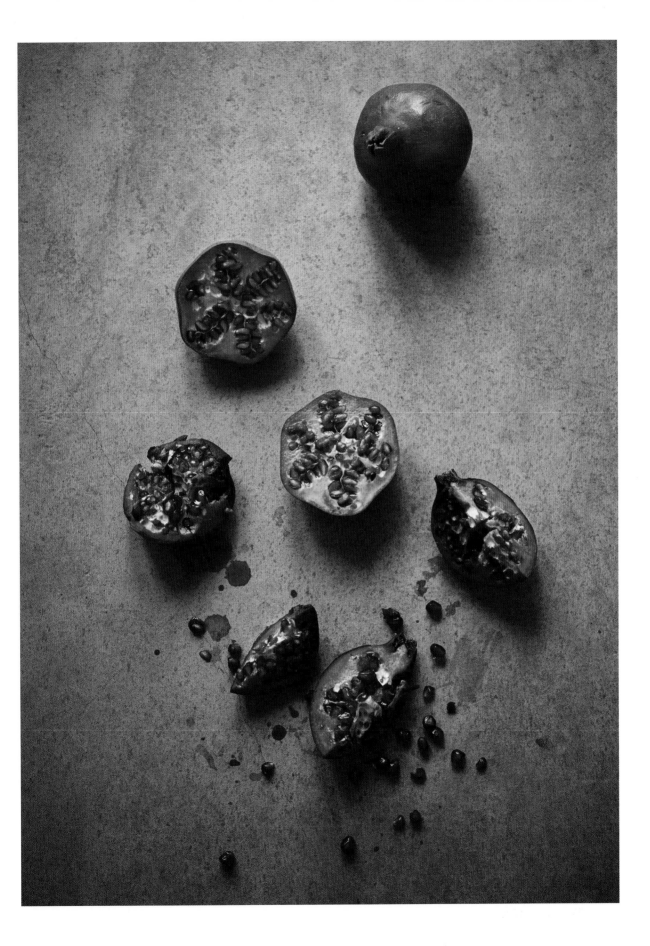

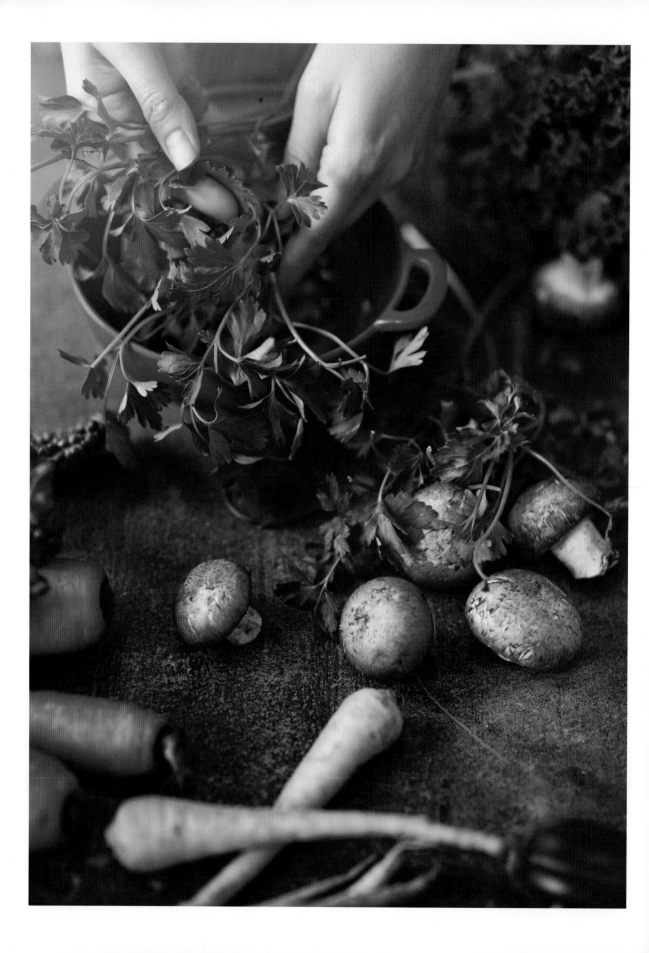

CHAPTER THREE

Functional and Dysfunctional Foods

Now that we've gone over the basics of nutrition, we want to bring all that information together for you. We've compiled a list of our most functional and dysfunctional foods. Functional foods contain all of those magical vitamins, minerals, phytonutrients, and antioxidants we've been talking about. They provide your body with nutritional support and enhance overall health by protecting your cells and helping you recover. Although there are many other nutrient-dense foods, these are some of the most important ones that we recommend you include in your diet as you go through treatment.

Dysfunctional foods, on the other hand, are the opposite of functional ones. They either harm the body or provide minimal nutritional support during cancer treatment. There are no hard-and-fast rules when it comes to foods you should absolutely eliminate, because each body is different and therefore has different needs, preferences, and requirements. Use our dysfunctional list only as a guide; if a food on this list beckons to you, use your judgment to assess if it's right for you to eat.

FUNCTIONAL FOODS TO EAT, EAT, EAT

CRUCIFEROUS VEGETABLES

Cruciferous vegetables include kale, cauliflower, cabbage, broccoli, broccoli sprouts, arugula, collards, Brussels sprouts, and bok choy. These vegetables are superfoods. They pack in a praiseworthy amount of vitamin A, vitamin C, and fiber, which all have their own unique ways of supporting immunity. Cruciferous veggies contain a significant amount of sulforaphane, indole-3-carbinol, and phenethyl isothiocyanate, phytonutrients that can inhibit the formation of tumors and suppress cell growth and metastasis. Sulforaphane specifically supports the detoxification pathway in the liver needed to process carcinogens and prevent the development of cancer. Indole-3-carbinol and a compound called diindolylmethane (DIM) have been found to prevent hormone-dominant cancers such as breast, endometrial, cervical, and prostate.

A quick note about supportive drugs during treatment: You may be placed on these kinds of medication to help with symptoms such as nausea, water retention, blood pressure, and blood clotting. Most of these drugs will not interact with the foods you eat. However, if you have been placed on warfarin (Coumadin), be mindful of your vitamin K intake—this mainly includes dark, leafy greens. If you're unsure of what to avoid or limit, talk to your doctor. You can always choose to remove the leafy greens from some of our recipes, like our smoothies, or focus on other delicious recipes that don't have greens.

MUSHROOMS

Mushrooms such as shiitake, enoki, cremini, portobello, chaga, oyster, turkey tail, reishi, and hen-of-the-woods have anticancer, antioxidant, prebiotic (a prebiotic is a type of fiber that feeds probiotics, the good bacteria in your digestive tract that support immunity), and anti-inflammatory properties. The antimicrobial properties in mushrooms means that they help fight off infections. Mushrooms have antitumor and immune-modulating effects. This means that mushrooms have the power to regulate your immune system, whether it needs to be suppressed or enhanced. Mushroom extracts can also reduce side effects of chemotherapy and radiation such as nausea, anemia, and bone marrow suppression. Certain complex carbs found mainly in mushrooms have been shown to make your immune cells respond faster, kill cancer cells, and inhibit metastasis. These mushrooms are widely used in Asia in combination with chemotherapy and radiation.

TURMERIC

Turmeric is a bright-yellow spice (fresh turmeric looks like an orange version of ginger root) that you'll find most commonly in powdered form. The healing compound in turmeric, curcumin, is responsible for turmeric's anticancer properties and has potent anti-inflammatory effects on your body. Studies show that curcumin, either alone or in combination with other drugs, increases tumor cell death in these cancers: brain, breast, ovarian, testicular, prostate, pancreatic, liver, colorectal, lung, lymphoma, leukemia, head and neck, bladder, and esophageal. Research also finds that curcumin can inhibit the growth of new blood vessels and suppress the proliferation of cancer cells. It's best to consume turmeric with a pinch of black pepper to increase its absorption in the body.

PROBIOTICS AND FERMENTED FOODS

A large part of your immune system (about 70–80 percent) is located in your gut. The digestive system is populated by a variety of microflora (made up of bacteria and yeasts) that regulate bowel movements, enhance nutrient absorption, and support immune function. Sometimes the microflora become unbalanced, a condition known as dysbiosis, which leaves the body compromised. Probiotics add good bacteria to the gut to help rebalance the population and fend off unwanted infections. This can be beneficial if you're suffering from digestive side effects of radiation or chemotherapy. Probiotics have antitumor effects, especially for colon, gastric, and bladder cancers. They also impact natural killer cells, which monitor the immune system against tumor development and infection. You will find probiotics in fermented foods like yogurt, kefir, sauerkraut, kimchi, kombucha, miso, tempeh, and in supplement form.

OMEGA-3 FATTY ACIDS

The most abundant sources of omega-3 fatty acids are fish oil, flax oil and seeds, chia seeds, salmon, trout, sardines, anchovies, herring, and mackerel. Studies show that omega-3 fatty acids affect cancer cell replication, cell cycle, and cell death and may sensitize tumors to anticancer drugs. Omega-3 fatty acids suppress inflammation and regulate cell signaling and gene expression, which play a role in cancer development. Cachexia, characterized by weight loss and muscle wasting, is one of the most severe side effects of cancer. Several studies of cachexic animals found that fish oil consumption led to increased body weight, improvement of white blood cell function, and prolonged survival. Omega-3 fatty acids might also improve effectiveness and tolerability of chemotherapy.

ALLIUM FAMILY

The allium family of vegetables includes garlic, onions, chives, scallions, shallots, and leeks. These vegetables all have antimicrobial, antitumor, and anticancer properties. Plants in the allium family contain organosulfur compounds, also present in cruciferous vegetables. These compounds are responsible for anticancer activity and have a hand in inducing cancer cell death. The allium family, especially garlic, improves detoxification in the liver, which helps neutralize, remove, and inhibit carcinogens and protect DNA from damage. These sulfur compounds protect you from carcinogens that are produced when meat is cooked at high temperatures while grilling or pan frying. Adding fresh or powdered onion and garlic to meat before cooking can help decrease carcinogen levels. The compounds in the allium family are especially beneficial to gastric and colon cancers.

BONE BROTH AND VEGETABLE BROTH

Bone and vegetable broths are both touted as health elixirs that help improve immunity. Broths made with animal bones contain gelatin, derived from collagen, and glycine, both of which help improve digestion by strengthening the intestinal lining and protecting against infection. This is important not only to enhance immunity, but also to help repair damage to the digestive system caused by cancer itself or by chemotherapy or radiation. Glycine also supports liver function so that it can detoxify chemotherapy drugs and other toxins and may reduce chemotherapy-induced liver damage.

The protein in bone broth is also helpful for muscle maintenance and growth, especially when muscle wasting as a result of treatment is a concern. The minerals found in bone and vegetable broths help replenish electrolytes that have been lost from vomiting, diarrhea, or sweat. Find our veggie and bone broth recipes in the soup section starting on page 115.

SOY

Soy and cancer have a controversial relationship. Most of the controversy is over the role of compounds called "isoflavones," which are a type of phytoestrogen that resembles estrogen. Phytoestrogens can bind to estrogen receptors in human cells and reduce the risk of cancer by blocking harmful forms of estrogen from binding. However, other studies suggest that soy protein can promote cancer cell growth. The issue here is with soy protein supplementation rather than eating whole foods made from soy. We recommend avoiding products that are processed and contain high amounts of isolated soy isoflavones, including soy flour, soy oil, and soy protein powder. These foods are not as healthy as whole-food sources of soy, such as tofu, tempeh, tamari, and miso, which are easier to digest.

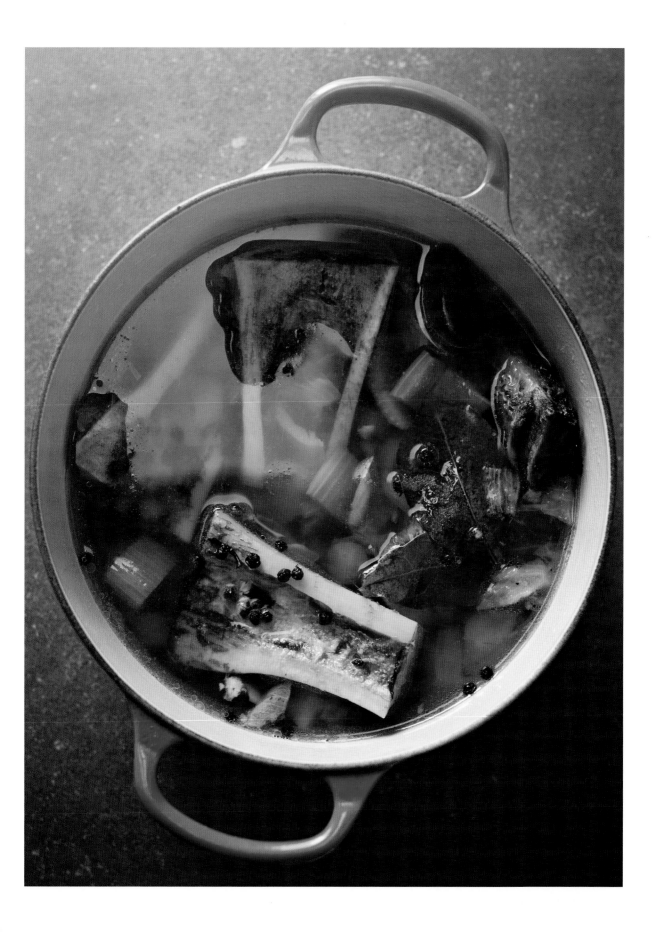

FRESH VEGGIE JUICES

Vegetable juices are easy to digest and provide nutrients that are absorbed immediately. Fresh juices can be very helpful if you are on a low-fiber diet or if you have trouble eating full meals due to cancer or treatment side effects. If you don't have a juicer, don't worry: there are juice bars that make fresh-pressed juices and even companies that can deliver fresh-pressed juices to you. Because juicing removes the fiber from the fruit or veggies, it's best to drink low-glycemic veggie juices that are made primarily from non-starchy vegetables such as leafy greens, cucumber, celery, and ginger, instead of all-fruit juices.

SUPER GREENS

Spirulina, chlorella, wheatgrass, and chlorophyll are super-potent greens that contain concentrated amounts of vitamins and minerals. Spirulina, a type of alga, has been found in studies to help prevent cancer cells from replicating. Chlorella, another type of alga, is a good source of omega-3 fatty acids and has been shown to improve quality of life in breast cancer patients, specifically by increasing energy. Studies have found that chlorella also has anticancer benefits and can induce cancer cell death and prevent DNA damage. Both spirulina and chlorella can be bought in tablets, to be swallowed with water, or in a powder that can be added to smoothies.

Wheatgrass is a green plant that is rich in minerals, vitamins, and chlorophyll, the pigment that gives plants their rich green color. You can also buy chlorophyll as a liquid supplement that can be added to water. Chlorophyll can help increase hemoglobin (the oxygen-carrying molecule) and red blood cells. Oxygen is vital for your cells to function optimally, and wheatgrass helps oxygenate cells and prevents cellular DNA damage. You can buy wheatgrass freeze-dried or freshly juiced at juice bars.

HERBS AND SPICES

Besides enhancing flavor and beautifying a plate, spices and herbs are valuable for your health and full of cancer-fighting properties. We recommend incorporating as many spices and herbs as you can into your diet during treatment and recovery. Here are some of our favorites.

- **Cloves** are antibacterial, antifungal, and antiviral.
- **Cumin** detoxifies carcinogens and prevents the growth of breast cancer cells.
- **Cinnamon** prevents tumor cells from growing and spreading and plays a role in promoting cancer cell death.
- **Ginger** helps ease nausea and has the ability to induce cancer cell death as well as prevent cancer cells from growing.
- **Parsley** is a powerful antioxidant that can protect cells from damage caused by carcinogens.
- **Rosemary** may prevent cancer cells from growing.

DYSFUNCTIONAL FOODS TO AVOID

RED MEAT AND PROCESSED MEAT

Red meat is linked with cancer in a variety of ways—one of them being its iron content, which may damage the lining of the colon and is associated with colon cancer. Other factors include its saturated fat content, its effect on insulin-like growth factors, and the formation of chemical compounds from high-heat cooking.

Processed meats, which are typically smoked, cured, and salted, contain nitrates. This is problematic because nitrates are precursors for the formation of carcinogens in the body. Grilling, barbecuing, high-heat cooking, and smoking meats also produces compounds that cause genetic mutations, and this plays a role in cancer development. You can decrease the amount of carcinogenic compounds produced by reducing the cooking temperature and the cooking time.

UNFERMENTED DAIRY

Consuming dairy during cancer is a controversial topic: there are many conflicting opinions and studies. Some studies show that dairy may reduce risk of certain cancers, like colorectal cancer, and other studies suggest it increases mortality and risk of prostate and breast cancers. It's been hypothesized that some cancers, like breast and prostate, are affected by dairy's saturated fat content, casein (its main protein), estrogenic hormones, and insulin-like growth factors (more on those below).

If you are going to eat dairy, sticking to fermented sources like yogurt and kefir is the best choice, since they both have positive probiotic effects. One of the main concerns with dairy and cancer development is that dairy increases the production of something called "insulin-like growth factor 1" (IGF-1). When IGF-1 circulates in the blood, it stimulates cancer cells to grow. It's also common for dairy to be difficult to digest, often due to its casein and lactose. During chemotherapy and radiation, digestion can be compromised, so it's important to eat foods that are easy on the stomach, rather than ones that pose challenges.

If you're going to eat dairy, opt for organic. The grains fed to conventional dairy cattle contain pesticide residue, which is then transferred into milk and other dairy products, along with antibiotics that the cows may have been given. Pesticides are known endocrine disruptors, meaning they disrupt or interfere with your reproductive, neurological, and hormonal health. We also recommend sheep's or goat's milk as an alternative to cow's milk, since it is easier to digest.

REFINED SUGAR AND REFINED GRAINS

Refined sugar and refined grains come in many forms: white sugar, cane sugar, evaporated cane sugar, raw sugar, brown sugar, corn syrup, high-fructose corn syrup, sucrose, fructose, white flour, and white rice. They are often found in bread, bagels, pretzels, pasta, crackers, cereal, tortillas, muffins, croissants, cookies, cake, donuts, packaged granola bars, and sugary drinks like soda and electrolyte drinks.

When undergoing treatment, the body is already compromised by cancer and treatment side effects, so it's essential that you avoid processed foods that can worsen nutrient deficiencies.

Refined sugars and grains are high glycemic (they raise blood sugar), and high-glycemic diets have been associated with risk of prostate, colon, breast, and pancreatic cancers. A study demonstrated that patients with stage three colon cancer who consumed more than two servings of a sugar-sweetened beverage a day had a significantly increased risk of cancer recurrence and mortality. A sugary diet can lead to insulin resistance and excess insulin circulating in the body, and this has been linked with increased cancer risk.

Refined sugars and grains also affect the gut's microflora. Much of the immune system sits within the gastrointestinal tract, and sugar promotes the overgrowth of unwanted bacteria. Simple sugars also compromise the body's ability to attack bad bacteria for up to five hours. This can compromise your body's immune system and contribute to unwanted inflammation.

ARTIFICIAL SWEETENERS

Artificial sweeteners may seem like a good alternative to refined sugar, but unfortunately they are not. These synthetic sweeteners seem like healthy alternatives because they lack calories, keep blood sugar balanced, and supposedly help with weight loss. You may know them by their brand names: Splenda, Sweet'n low, Sugar Twin, NutraSweet, NatraTaste, and Equal, but they're also found in lots of food products, medicines, and dental hygiene items. There have been many studies over the years that show evidence (or not) of the carcinogenicity of artificial sweeteners. The truth is these sweeteners actually cause people to crave more sweets and find naturally sweet foods unpalatable due to changes in their taste buds. We need long-term studies to truly understand the impact of these artificial sweeteners on health and especially on cancer development. So in the meantime, we recommend avoiding them.

NATURAL SWEETENERS

Although they are in our "dysfunctional foods" list, we often use small quantities of natural sweeteners, like pure maple syrup, honey, brown rice syrup, molasses, dates and date syrup, coconut sugar, and coconut sap in our recipes. They do still function similarly to sugar, because they break down quickly and spike your blood sugar, but these sweeteners also have benefits beyond just being sweet, like not being artificially made and containing vitamins and minerals.

ALCOHOL

Alcohol consumption has long been associated with cancer risk and mortality. The exact mechanism of how alcohol increases cancer risk is still being researched, but here's what we know: when alcohol is broken down in the liver, a toxic substance called acetaldehyde is created, and this is believed to cause DNA damage. While undergoing cancer treatment, the liver works hard to detoxify everyday substances, including hormones like estrogen, and has the additional burden of chemotherapy drugs and possible radiation exposure. Alcohol burdens the liver, can damage liver cells, and create inflammation, affecting overall liver function and its ability to detoxify substances properly. Your liver is important during treatment, so we highly recommend avoiding alcohol.

VEGETABLE OILS

The most common cooking oils are vegetable oils, including soy, corn, canola, and safflower. Vegetable oil is relatively inexpensive, and it is shelf- and heat-stable because it's heavily refined, bleached, deodorized, and possibly hydrogenated to appear translucent, with no real detectable taste or smell. While this may seem ideal for cooking or baking, it's not ideal for your health. Processing vegetable oil removes all the nutritious benefits, and the oils are heated to such high temperatures in the deodorizing phase that the beneficial fatty acids in the oils become mutagenic and promote inflammation. Without any vitamins or minerals, vegetable oil is equivalent to white sugar and white flour.

Flip back a few pages, to pages 16–17, to find out which oils are best for you to use.

Let's Talk about Intuitive Eating

Most of the time only you know best what your body needs. Yes, YOU! Intuitive eating means paying attention to your cravings, your aversions, and really to what your "gut" is telling you. By "your gut" we mean two things: "I have a gut feeling," and at the same time your gut as in your gastrointestinal tract. Sometimes cravings, like ones for sugar, happen because the harmful bacteria in your gut are desperate for sugar to help them grow. Or you might feel sad or tired, so you crave sugar to make yourself feel better—but it only works momentarily.

We call this a "surface craving," and this is one you want to do your absolute best not to give in to. A surface craving is usually not going to provide you or your body with any real nutrition. If you wait, these cravings tend to go away within ten to fifteen minutes. You also know that you may feel unwell, bloated, or guilty after eating these types of foods. A "deep craving," on the other hand, is one that your body is screaming for because it may want the nutrients from a particular food. For example, if you're craving sweet potatoes, maybe your body needs the beta-carotene, healthy complex carbohydrates, fiber, or even the energetic, grounding and earthy qualities that sweet potatoes offer.

While undergoing cancer treatment, your appetite changes, so sometimes when you do finally feel hungry and you actually have a craving you want to immediately fulfill it. We think this is so important, but (yes there's a but) check in with yourself first. For instance, if your appetite reemerges and you want a burger and fries, well, we know that a white bun is made from nonnutritious white flour, red meat may promote tumor growth, and fries are heated in toxic oils (did we just ruin this for you?). So check in with yourself to see if this is a surface craving, a deep craving, or what your body really *needs*. Sometimes this is a deep craving and your body wants the protein and fat from a beef burger, and sometimes it's a surface craving because eating a burger is comforting and reminds you of your childhood.

What we mean to say is that *you* have the answers. Even though foods may be on our functional or dysfunctional food lists, *you* truly know what's best for *you*. If you are craving something that you know is not healthful for you, try to make alternatives (many are found in this very cookbook) and see if that satisfies you. Take our information, use it, study it; make our recipes; and then continue to ask yourself, "What food will nourish my body today?" If you're unsure how to decipher what your body really needs, we suggest sitting quietly for three minutes, paying attention to your inhales and exhales and continuing to ask yourself, "What do I need?" This may seem awkward at first, but you will get the hang of it and some important information may present itself. If it doesn't, well, hey, you just meditated for three minutes and that's a pretty good thing too!

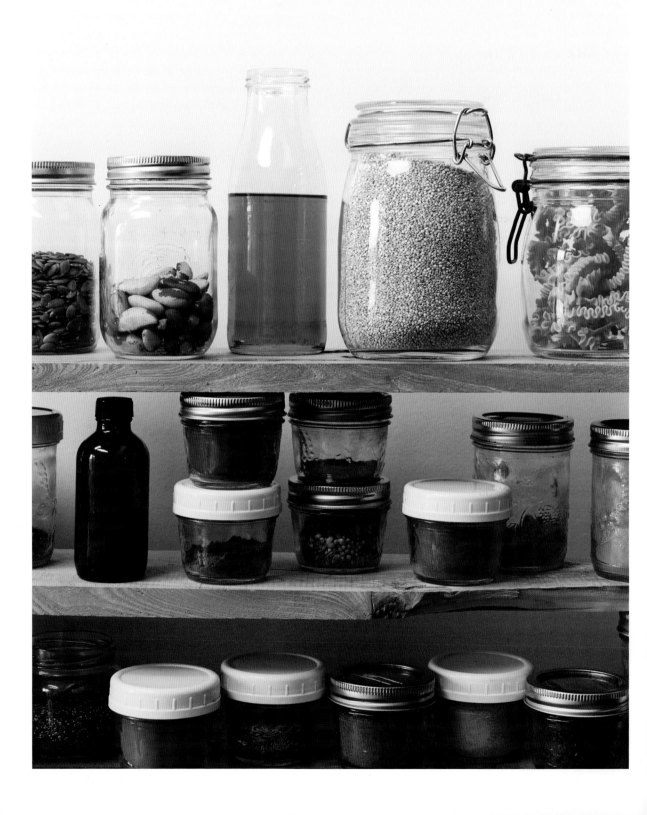

CHAPTER FOUR

Eating to Combat Common Side Effects

It can be daunting to figure out what you should be eating before, during, and after treatment. When undergoing cancer therapies, your experiences may feel all over the map: one day you may be nauseated with no appetite, and the next day you may feel energetic and hungry. We're going to address what to do when you experience side effects. If you're unsure where to start, what to eat, and which recipes to choose, use our menu plans as your guide. We have created a multitude of recipes that include powerhouse ingredients to work *with* your body, rather than *against* it.

A NOTE ABOUT OUR MENU PLANS

The menu plans below are laid out with different recipes for each day. Dinner leftovers are meant to be eaten as lunch the next day to save time and avoid cooking additional meals. You can also cook large batches of one meal and eat that throughout the week. If these plans are too overwhelming, we welcome you to simplify them. Use them as your guide and make it work for you and your needs.

WHAT TO EAT BEFORE TREATMENT

Before you actually begin treatment you may be feeling fine, or you may be dealing with painful symptoms. Regardless, this is the time to amp up your nutrition and eat as cleanly as possible, especially while your appetite is still intact and strong.

It's important to support your immune system and your detoxification organs like your colon, your liver, and your kidneys. Treatments can be quite aggressive and are designed to decrease immunity. Think of this time as the training period before the event: you need to strengthen your body and have a good store of nutrients so that when it's time to undergo therapies, you'll be in a nourished state and better able to handle treatment.

IMMUNE-SUPPORTIVE FOODS

You want to be as healthy as possible when going to the hospital for treatment so that your body is not compromised by fighting off bacteria, viruses, or infections at the same time as facing treatment. Eat immune-supportive foods like onions, garlic, ginger, lemons, blueberries, kale, broccoli, and turmeric.

REDUCE SUGAR INTAKE

Sugar can interfere with your white blood cell function for up to five hours after ingestion. Focus on eating foods that will keep your blood sugar stable and your insulin levels lower, like whole grains, beans, vegetables, and healthy proteins.

HEALTHY FATS AND PROTEIN

Eating healthy fats and protein will strengthen your body so that you don't feel weak going into treatment. Eat avocado, seeds, and nuts or put a tablespoon of coconut oil, flax oil, or hemp oil into your smoothies.

AVOID PRO-INFLAMMATORY FOODS

Avoid eating pro-inflammatory foods like processed meat, alcohol, soda, baked goods, most commercially made snacks, chips, vegetable oils (canola, soy, corn, sunflower, and safflower), sugar, refined flour, processed and deep-fried foods, and gluten if you are sensitive to it. We also recommend limiting red meat and unfermented dairy. Avoid cooking at high temperatures, especially above 400°F, and never reuse cooking oil.

AVOID EATING YOUR FAVORITE FOODS THE DAY BEFORE TREATMENT

On the day of treatment or the days following you may feel unwell. Usually people remember the foods they ate right before getting sick and then can develop a negative, visceral reaction to the thought of eating those foods in the future. If you can, try to reserve your favorites for when you are feeling better or when treatment is over.

It's best to eat foods that are simple the day before treatment. Avoid anything that has intense flavors or spices, and avoid foods that are heavy or difficult to digest. Easy smoothies, oatmeal, soup, steamed greens, eggs, and mashed veggies are all great options.

DRINK MORE WATER

Make sure to drink lots of fluids to help your body remove waste and hydrate before treatment. Aim to drink about two quarts, or six to eight cups, of water a day.

PRE-TREATMENT MENU PLAN

	DAY 1	DAY 2	DAY 3	DAY 4	DAY 5
Breakfast	Pesto Vegetable Quiche* (page 109)	Cinnamon Quinoa Breakfast Bowl (page 101)	Pesto Vegetable Quiche* (page 109)	Dulse, Egg, and Avocado Special (page 103)	Classic Granola (page 98)
Juice/ Smoothie/Elixir	Starter Green smoothie (page 74)	Miracle Matcha Latte (page 91)	Broccoli Pear juice (page 85)	Olympic Gold Milk (page 90)	Superfood Beet smoothie (page 77)
Lunch	Salsa-Stuffed Avocado (page 173) + Over the Rainbow Slaw* (page 188)	Pesto Sweet Potato Chicken Salad* (page 136) + Loaded Vegetable Salad* (page 186)	Black Bean Tex Mex Burgers* (page 156) + Over the Rainbow Slaw (page 188)	Rustic Salsa Trout (page 145) + Emerald-Green Garlic Sauté* (page 183)	Middle Eastern Spiced Chicken* (page 146) + Colorful Root Fries (page 191)
Snack	Organic Chicken Broth** (page 118) or Phyto Broth** (page 119)	Chickpea Popkins* (page 222)	Organic Chicken Broth** (page 118) or Phyto Broth** (page 119)	Sunflower Hummus + veggie sticks (page 206)	Chickpea Popkins* (page 222)
Dinner	Pesto Sweet Potato Chicken Salad* (page 136) + Loaded Vegetable Salad* (page 186)	Black Bean Tex Mex Burgers* (page 156) + Over the Rainbow Slaw (page 188)	Rustic Salsa Trout (page 145) + Emerald-Green Garlic Sauté* (page 183)	Middle Eastern Spiced Chicken* (page 146) + Colorful Root Fries (page 191)	Chutney and Coconut Red Lentil Soup** (page 132)

* These recipes make several portions, so it's a good idea to make these items in advance and then use them for multiple meals.

** We recommend preparing these recipes in advance, before your treatment. Make larger batches of soups and stews and then freeze them so it's easy to defrost and reheat them when you aren't feeling well.

WHAT TO PREPARE BEFORE TREATMENT TO EAT AFTER TREATMENT

Prepare this food in advance, to eat during treatment or after treatment when you don't have the energy or feel well enough to cook. Caregivers and loved ones, this is a great time for you to step in.

Whether you are cooking for yourself or for a loved one, it is best to make as many items as possible in advance so that you don't have to think about cooking or preparing food when you aren't feeling well.

BROTHS AND SOUPS

Prepare a nutrient-rich vegetable broth, bone broth, or chicken broth (check out our chapter on soups). Even if you can't eat food for the first few days after treatment, sipping a nourishing broth will keep you hydrated and provide your body with important minerals. Bone broth is rich in gelatin, strengthening the intestinal lining and helping the liver detoxify.

To make soup or broth more appetizing and easier to eat, slowly sip it from a mug rather than serving it in a large bowl.

Soups and broths are freezer friendly, so they are some of the best recipes to make in advance, freeze, and heat up when you need them most. You'll find instructions on freezing soups in the recipes.

ELECTROLYTE DRINKS

After treatment, you may become dehydrated, either because you're not drinking enough or because you are experiencing side effects like vomiting or diarrhea. You'll need to replenish your electrolytes. Drink coconut water or make our Energizing Electrolyte Drink (page 87).

SMOOTHIES

Smoothies can replace normal meals when eating is a challenge, and they can help prevent weight and muscle loss. The best way to prep smoothies in advance is to make a bunch of smoothie packs. Chop and measure out all of the ingredients, except for the liquid, and store them in airtight ziplock bags or containers in the freezer. Then, when you are ready to make a smoothie, throw the smoothie pack into the blender with some liquid and whip it up in less than a minute. You can find our smoothie recipes starting on page 71.

EASY-TO-EAT VEGETABLES

Soft, pureed, and mashed vegetables are much easier to eat than raw vegetables and are more palatable if you feel nauseated or lack an appetite. Some of our side dish recipes, pages 178–199, blend veggies together or cook them well so they're soft and easy to chew and eat. You can easily freeze cooked veggies and reheat them in the oven when you're ready to eat.

VEGETARIAN AND OMNIVORE MAINS

Our main dishes freeze incredibly well and can quickly and easily be defrosted. It's best to freeze them in smaller portions, so that if your appetite isn't strong, you can defrost a small serving and prevent wasting any food.

BLAND AND DRY FOODS

Crackers and biscuits are generally easier than other foods to eat when you feel nauseated or sick. Spreading a little butter, ghee, nut or seed butter, coconut oil, or coconut butter on top adds extra fat, for more energy. We have recipes for these in the snacks chapter (page 201). It's best to make these before going into treatment so you have them on hand afterward.

WARMING BEVERAGES

Our elixirs are a good way to soothe your body, support relaxation, and even help combat nausea. You may become sensitive to temperature and find it easier to drink something warm instead of cold or at room temperature.

VEGETABLE JUICES

If you have a juicer or even a high-speed blender, making fresh veggie juice is a wonderful way to ensure you are getting nutrients without needing to eat a full meal. Find our juice recipes starting on page 81.

SAUCES, MARINADES, AND DRESSINGS

It's helpful to have a few different sauces, marinades, and dressings prepared and stored in the fridge before treatment begins. This makes it easy to quickly add extra flavor and seasoning to simple meals when you aren't feeling well or don't want to cook.

WHAT TO EAT ON TREATMENT DAYS

Caregivers, if your loved one is an inpatient, you can bring these items to them.

Although treatment days may be the most challenging because of anxiety, stress, or discomfort from side effects, we encourage you to prepare and bring food with you on these days, even if you don't end up eating everything. Prep and pack your snacks and meals in advance, a day or two before, so that you don't have to think about organizing anything on the actual day of treatment.

LIGHT SNACKS

Healthy crackers, granola bars, and muffins are all good options, as they're not as heavy and difficult to eat as full meals. For more light snacks, flip to page 201. You can bring simple, easy-to-digest foods like cooked vegetables and brown rice to keep your energy up.

FLUIDS

Drink water throughout the day, when you can, to prevent dehydration. It's helpful if you add some electrolyte powder to your water bottle, or drink coconut water or our Energizing Electrolyte Drink (page 87). You can also bring a thermos of broth, soup, or stew, or a jar with a smoothie or some juice with you for added hydration and nutrition.

GRAB-AND-GO FOODS

Grab-and-go's are foods that you can eat with your hands and that are good cold, warm, hot, or at room temperature. They provide a significant amount of nutrition and energy to the body. Some examples of these foods are veggie burgers, chicken fingers, muffins, and our Power Truffles (page 213).

DURING-TREATMENT MENU PLAN

The during-treatment menu plan is for when you're experiencing side effects. We've chosen to structure this menu plan differently from the other ones in this section. Instead of labeling meals as breakfast, lunch, and dinner, we suggest foods you can eat at any time of the day depending on how you feel. If you need a light or liquid meal because you're unable to eat heavier, substantial dishes, this is where you turn. This plan includes recipes that are easy to digest, easy to eat, and easy to swallow, and ideal for when you are experiencing side effects.

	DAY 1	DAY 2	DAY 3	DAY 4	DAY 5
Light Meal	Chia Coconut Breakfast Pudding* (page 112)	Blended Berry smoothie (page 79)	Chia Coconut Breakfast Pudding* (page 112)	Overnight Oats* (page 111)	Overnight Oats* (page 111)
Nutrient Drinks	Fresh Ginger Tea (page 93)	Olympic Gold Milk (page 90)	Immunity Zip juice (page 86)	Kickstarter Kale juice (page 83)	Energizing Electrolyte Drink (page 87)
Liquid Snack/ Meal	Broth of choice (Chicken, Bone, Phyto)** (page 118–120)	Restore smoothie (page 74)	Soothing Squash Ginger Soup** (page 123)	Greena Colada smoothie (page 78)	Broccoli Coconut Soup** (page 124)
Snacks	Immune-Boosting Applesauce** (page 221)	Coconut Flour Biscuits* (with butter for extra calories) (page 215)	Lemon Ginger Fat Bombs (page 219)	Coconut Flour Biscuits* (with butter for extra calories) (page 215)	Zesty Blueberry Granola Bars (page 209)*
Soft Vegetables	Sautéed Mushrooms over Sweet Potato Mash (page 189)	Turnip Beet Mash* (page 197)	Indian Spiced Popcorn Cauliflower* (page 192)	Spiced Sweet Potato Wedges (page 198)	Indian Spiced Popcorn Cauliflower* (page 192)
Travel-Friendly Foods	Grain-Free Farinata Flatbread* (page 203)	Superfood Trail Mix* (page 207)	Apple Cinnamon Muffins* (page 210)	Superfood Trail Mix* (page 207)	Power Truffles* (page 213)
Meals	Ayurvedic Kichadi** (page 167)	Lentil Shepherd's Pie* (page 171)	Ayurvedic Kichadi** (page 167)	Turkey White Bean Stew* (page 140)	Stewed Coconut, Tomato, and Chickpeas** (page 162)

* These recipes make several portions, so it's a good idea to make these items in advance and then use them for multiple meals.

** We recommend preparing these recipes in advance, before your treatment. Make larger batches of soups and stews and then freeze them so it's easy to defrost and reheat them when you aren't feeling well.

DEALING WITH SIDE EFFECTS

Before reading this section, please note that everyone has a unique experience dealing with side effects. Cancer treatment impacts cells that are dividing quickly, and cancer cells replicate at a much faster rate than normal cells. The digestive system, bone marrow, hair, and skin have cells that replicate and repair more frequently than other areas of the body. This makes healthy cells in these areas more susceptible to damage caused by chemotherapy and radiation, which is one of the reasons it is common to experience side effects like nausea, vomiting, mouth sores, and hair loss.

We'll outline what side effects may occur and suggest different foods and techniques to help combat them. Our goal is to support you nutritionally so that your body is in the best state to recover quickly from treatment. If you experience any of the following side effects, do your best to keep your caloric intake up and stay hydrated.

≋ NAUSEA AND VOMITING

Many people tend to feel nauseated immediately after treatment, and this may last until the next day or even for a few days afterward. Staying hydrated during this time is vital in order to prevent dehydration. Here are suggestions to help.

- Drink broth and simple soup.
- Eat dry, bland foods such as crackers and biscuits.
- Drink one of our warming elixirs, or ginger or peppermint tea.
- Drink our Energizing Electrolyte Drink (page 87) or coconut water.
- Eat small snacks more frequently, as an empty stomach can make nausea worse.
- Avoid heavy, oily, fried, or spicy foods.

Top Recipes to Help with Nausea
- Rosemary Currant Hazelnut Crackers (page 204)
- Coconut Flour Biscuits (page 215)
- Organic Chicken Broth (page 118), Strong Bones Broth (page 120), or Phyto Broth (page 119)
- Hydrating Ginger Lemonade (page 88)
- Fresh Ginger Tea (page 93)
- Energizing Electrolyte Drink (page 87)

We eat with our eyes first, and a big plate of food can be overwhelming if you have no appetite. It's still essential that you eat something, so try using smaller dishes, like salad plates, mugs, or bowls, to serve smaller portions of food. You'll want to focus on eating "bang for your buck" foods, meaning high-calorie and nutritious items, to make sure you get more nutrients when you are able to eat.

- Drink a glass of lemon water to stimulate digestive juices. Squeeze a quarter of a fresh lemon into a cup of warm water. It's best to drink lemon water first thing in the morning or about ten to fifteen minutes before eating a meal.
- Try taking half a teaspoon of apple cider vinegar in a small glass of water ten minutes before a meal to stimulate appetite.
- Avoid drinking liquids during meals, to prevent feeling full while eating.
- Try eating cold, warm, and hot foods and see which temperature is most appealing to you.
- Eat simple foods that are high in calories and nutrients, like smoothies and our snack recipes.
- Eat bitter foods like rapini and turmeric to stimulate appetite.

Top Recipes to Help with Loss of Appetite
- Superfood Trail Mix (page 207)
- Organic Chicken Broth (page 118), Phyto Broth (page 119), or Strong Bones Broth (page 120)
- Power Truffles (page 213)
- Garlic Rapini with Sundried Tomatoes (page 194)
- Gingersnap Cookies (page 233)
- Olympic Gold Milk (page 90)

Many cancer treatments impact taste, smell, and saliva production. You may experience that foods start to taste metallic, like cardboard, or just bland. This can be frustrating, especially if you are unable to taste flavors that you typically enjoy. Here are some tips to combat these particular side effects.

- If you experience a metallic taste in your mouth, try eating with plastic cutlery.
- Rinse out your mouth before and after meals with warm salt water (avoid this tip if you have mouth sores, as salt water will aggravate them).
- Add extra herbs to meals, for example, parsley, basil, dill, cilantro, thyme, rosemary, or oregano.
- Add spices to enhance the flavor of dishes, for example, cumin, cinnamon, coriander, sumac, za'atar, chili powder, and paprika.
- Try cuisines like Moroccan, Mediterranean, Indian, or Thai, which incorporate lots of spices and flavors your taste buds may not be used to.
- Add fresh garlic or roasted garlic to savory meals to bring out flavor.
- If foods tastes metallic, add a bit of acid over top—for instance, lemon juice, lime juice, or orange juice.
- If food tastes bland and dry, add sea salt or drizzle oil (extra-virgin olive oil, flax oil, hemp oil, or coconut oil) over your meal.
- If food tastes bitter, add sweeter vegetables (sweet potatoes, squash, or carrots) or sweet fruits (berries, dates, bananas, or mango).
- Eat food at cooler temperatures or room temperature to reduce strong smells.

Top Recipes to Help Altered Taste or Smell
- Lemon Custard (page 237)
- Toasted Sesame Arame and Carrot Kale Sauté (page 178)
- Middle Eastern Spiced Chicken (page 146)
- Ayurvedic Kichadi (page 167)
- Saag Coconut Chicken (page 143)
- Hempy Pesto (page 243)

◆ DRY MOUTH (XEROSTOMIA)

Along with altered taste, it is common to experience reduced saliva production. This can make it difficult to chew, swallow, and enjoy many foods, especially if they are on the drier side. If you're experiencing dry mouth, focus on eating foods that contain moisture. You can also try the following.

- Make lots of extra sauce and dressing and pour it over meals, especially drier dishes.
- Stay hydrated and drink lots of water.
- Drizzle extra oil, like extra-virgin olive oil, flax oil, hemp oil, or coconut oil, over foods.
- Swish a teaspoon of coconut oil around in your mouth before eating to lubricate it (swish for at least a minute).
- Eat more liquid meals, like soup, broth, stew, smoothies, and juices.
- Avoid dry muffins, breads, and cookies.
- Avoid excess salt and spicy foods, as these can dehydrate the mouth more.
- Avoid caffeine (coffee, soda, and black tea). It is a diuretic and promotes the loss of fluid.

Top Recipes to Help Dry Mouth
- Creamy Tomato Soup (page 126)
- Broccoli Coconut Soup (page 124)
- Turnip Beet Mash (page 197)
- Chia Coconut Breakfast Pudding (page 112)
- Flax Oil Anti-Inflammation Dressing (page 250)
- Avocado Chocolate Mousse (page 231)

During treatment, sores may form on the lips, tongue, gums, or inside of the cheeks. They can be very painful and they often feel like a burn. It's very important to eat well when you have mouth sores, because when the cells in the mouth are damaged from treatment, your body's immune system is compromised as well.

- Eat soft, cooked foods such as mashed vegetables and chia pudding (page 112).
- Add extra non-acid-based sauce or dressing to your meals.
- Drink smoothies (page 71).
- Drink broths and blended soups (page 115).
- Cut your food into small pieces.
- Avoid extremely hot or cold foods if they cause irritation.
- Avoid spicy, acidic, and very salty foods, as these can be irritating.
- Swish a teaspoon of coconut oil around in your mouth every morning to lubricate it (swish for at least a minute).

Top Recipes to Help with Sore Mouth
- Turnip Beet Mash (page 197)
- Chia Coconut Breakfast Pudding (page 112)
- Overnight Oats (page 111)
- Cacao Fat Bombs (page 219)
- Soothing Squash Ginger Soup (page 123)
- Avocado Chocolate Mousse (page 231)

◊ DIFFICULTY SWALLOWING (DYSPHAGIA)

Difficulty swallowing can be caused by swelling, or inflammation of the cells lining the esophagus and throat, or by low saliva production. You may find talking difficult, or you may find that it feels as if food gets stuck in your throat. You may also feel the need to cough, or feel a gag reflex when eating.

- Cut food into small pieces or puree to make it easier to eat.
- Focus on liquids, such as smoothies, juices, soups, and broths.
- Add extra sauce and dressings to your meals to lubricate them.
- Eat cooked soft foods and mashed foods (such as squash and sweet potato), as they are easier to swallow.
- Avoid extremely hot food temperatures and spicy foods because they may be irritating.
- Limit or avoid acidic foods such as citrus, tomatoes, and pineapple if you find them irritating.

Top Recipes to Help with Swallowing
- All smoothies (page 71)
- Immune-Boosting Applesauce (page 221)
- Chutney and Coconut Red Lentil Soup (page 132)
- Organic Chicken Broth (page 118), Phyto Broth (page 119), and Strong Bones Broth (page 120)
- Miracle Matcha Latte (page 91)
- Overnight Oats (page 111)

DIARRHEA AND CONSTIPATION

It's common to experience diarrhea and constipation when the cells of the gastrointestinal tract are damaged from treatment or medication. Fiber is often recommended to help both diarrhea and constipation; however, it is extremely important to eat the right type of fiber. Soluble fiber found in foods like ground flaxseeds, chia seeds, and cooked root vegetables can help. Insoluble fiber, found in leafy greens, celery, fruit, and beans, may be more irritating if you're struggling with diarrhea, though it can be helpful for constipation as it helps bulk up the stool and eliminate it from the body. It's best to limit non-starchy vegetables and leafy greens when dealing with diarrhea.

Staying hydrated is important to prevent dehydration if you have diarrhea and to help loosen stools if you have constipation. Electrolytes also play a role in normalizing stool consistency, so if you're dealing with diarrhea, drinking electrolytes will help replace the nutrients that are being lost too quickly. And if you're constipated, electrolytes will help your intestinal muscles work properly.

Ⓓ DIARRHEA

- Drink water and electrolytes to counter fluid loss.
- Avoid raw vegetables.
- Avoid dairy products because dairy can be irritating.
- Try eating bananas, rice, applesauce, and toast to help ease diarrhea.
- Eat probiotic foods like kombucha, dairy-free coconut yogurt, and sauerkraut to support a healthy balance of gut microflora.
- Eat soothing cooked foods such as soup, broth, and stew.
- Soluble fiber, such as ground flaxseeds, chia seeds, and oats, can help bulk up stool.

Top Recipes to Help with Diarrhea
- Healing Miso Soup (page 121)
- Energizing Electrolyte Drink (page 87)
- Organic Chicken Broth (page 118), Phyto Broth (page 119), or Strong Bones Broth (page 120)
- Chia Coconut Breakfast Pudding (page 112)
- Deep Green and Clean juice (page 85)

- Increase water and fluid intake, as well as electrolytes.
- Try drinking one cup of water with one to two tablespoons of fresh lemon juice first thing in the morning.
- Eat leafy greens and fibrous vegetables such as celery, kale, collards, broccoli, and spinach.
- Increase soluble fiber intake such as chia seeds, ground flaxseeds, and oats.
- Eat probiotic foods like kombucha, dairy-free coconut yogurt, and sauerkraut to support a healthy balance of gut microflora.

Top Recipes to Help with Constipation
- Energizing Electrolyte Drink (page 87)
- Loaded Vegetable Salad (page 186)
- Garlic Rapini with Sundried Tomatoes (page 194)
- Chia Coconut Breakfast Pudding (page 112)
- Rainbow Wraps (page 161)

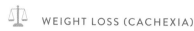 WEIGHT LOSS (CACHEXIA)

Weight loss is a common side effect that many people experience when undergoing cancer treatment. This is caused by low appetite or even the cancer itself. Our recipes work to prevent weight loss, as it can be challenging to maintain energy and strength when your weight is compromised.

- Drink high-calorie smoothies and eat our healthy desserts.
- Eat snacks between meals to keep blood sugar balanced.
- Try to eat protein and carbohydrates together—for example, an apple with almond butter or healthy crackers with hummus.
- Add extra healthy fats to your diet: drizzle or spread extra-virgin olive oil, coconut oil, coconut butter, hemp oil, flax oil, ghee, or butter onto meals or snacks whenever possible.
- Snack on nuts, seeds, nut or seed butter, and avocados.
- Eat low-glycemic, healthy carbohydrates, such as whole grains (brown rice, quinoa, millet, oats) and root vegetables (sweet potatoes, squash, beets, parsnips) to make sure your body has enough fuel and doesn't burn your fat stores for energy.
- Eat our omnivore or vegetarian mains for higher macronutrient intake.
- If you are doing any physical activity, always eat carbohydrates and protein to replenish.

Top Recipes to Help with Weight Loss
- Restore smoothie (page 74)
- Silver Dollar Vanilla Pancakes (page 104)
- Cacao Fat Bombs (page 219)
- Apple Cinnamon Muffins (page 210)
- Salsa-Stuffed Avocado (page 173)
- Turkey White Bean Stew (page 140)

Cancer and cancer treatments can make you feel very tired, lethargic, unmotivated, and weak. The best way to help your fatigue is to get as much rest as possible, take big, deep breaths throughout the day, drink lots of water, exercise when you can, and eat foods that are easy to digest and offer your body a lot of energy. You may not feel up to cooking, so when you have a surge of energy, make large batches of meals, snacks, and soups and freeze them so that they'll be there when you need them.

- Drink green juice and smoothies. They deliver nutrition quickly, and your body does not need to work hard to digest and assimilate the nutrients.
- Focus on eating easy-to-prepare foods, like smoothies, snacks, and soups.
- Eat foods that were prepared in advance and stored in the freezer.
- Make sure to eat healthy proteins and fats like nuts, seeds, legumes, fish, chicken, and eggs to support healing and repair of the body.
- Eat lots of produce that is rich in vitamin C, like leafy greens, bell peppers, root veggies, oranges, and lemons.
- Eat whole grains that are rich in B vitamins, like quinoa and brown rice.
- Stay hydrated, and add electrolytes, chlorophyll, and lemon juice to your water for extra boosts.

Top Recipe to Help with Exhaustion and Fatigue
- Pesto Vegetable Quiche (page 109)
- Turkey White Bean Stew (page 140)
- Healthy Ramen soup (page 129)
- Kickstarter Kale juice (page 83)
- Pesto Sweet Potato Chicken Salad (page 136)
- Miracle Matcha Latte (page 91)

People often focus on the physical challenges that come from treatment, yet the mental and emotional side effects are just as significant. Many people undergoing cancer treatment experience depression and anxiety, and we believe food can help. Ninety percent of serotonin, the feel-good, happy chemical, is actually made in the gut, so supporting healthy digestion is important for producing it.

- Eat foods rich in B_{12} and vitamin D, like tuna, salmon, cod, liver, yogurt, and shiitake mushrooms.
- Stand out in the sun for fifteen minutes, sit by a window, or get a light-therapy lamp.
- Eat selenium-rich foods, like brazil nuts, salmon, cod, tuna, chicken, turkey, eggs, tahini, and sunflower seeds.
- Eat omega-3-rich fish, hemp seeds, and flaxseeds.
- Raw cacao and dark chocolate (85 percent cacao) contain magnesium and tryptophan, which help relax the body and produce serotonin.
- Eat probiotic foods to maintain the integrity of the gut, like sauerkraut, tempeh, miso, and kimchi.
- Surround yourself with people you love and who uplift you.
- Practice happiness meditations, listen to uplifting music, and recite positive affirmations.
- Be physically active to the best of your ability. Even short walks count.

Top Recipes to Help with Depression and Anxiety
- Organic Chicken Broth (page 118), Phyto Broth (page 119), or Strong Bones Broth (page 120)
- Chocolate Almond smoothie (page 76)
- Avocado Chocolate Mousse (page 231)
- Dill Salmon Burgers (page 149)
- Classic Granola (page 98)

WHAT TO EAT IN REMISSION

At this point you may have more strength and have regained an appetite. This is the time to support your body back to health. Eat foods that help detoxify radiation, as well as chemotherapy and any other medications from your body. It is also essential to focus on eating foods that will strengthen your healthy cells and help your body repair damage.

LIVER-SUPPORTING FOODS

Your liver function is incredibly important when it comes to preventing and recovering from cancer. All substances—food, chemotherapy drugs, pesticides, cosmetics, hormones, household cleaners, pollution, and perfume—must be filtered by your liver in order to be removed from the body. Supporting this organ through diet is a safe and effective way to help it work optimally so that it can properly metabolize and remove toxins, which is especially important if you're in remission or between treatment cycles.

Here are the best foods to support the liver:
- bitter veggies, like arugula, rapini, and kale
- cruciferous veggies, like broccoli, cauliflower, Brussels sprouts, cabbage, and kale
- beets
- lemons
- onions, leeks, green onions, and garlic
- turmeric
- bone broth

CELL-SUPPORTING FOODS

Although cancer treatments like chemotherapy and radiation kill off cancer cells, they also cause damage to healthy cells. After treatment, it is vital to eat foods that support the body's cells, so that toxins from treatment can be removed, and healthy cells can strengthen and rebuild. This also helps prevent abnormal cells and cancer growth from recurring.

Here are the best foods to support healthy cells:

- super greens, like chlorophyll, spirulina, chlorella, and wheatgrass
- fermented foods such as sauerkraut, kimchi, kefir, yogurt, miso, and tempeh
- seaweeds, like arame, nori, and dulse
- turmeric

Find these important nutrients in the following foods:

- coenzyme Q10: salmon, sardines, liver, quinoa, millet, and rice
- selenium: Brazil nuts, salmon, mushrooms, turkey, cod, chicken, lamb, and eggs
- beta-carotene: carrots, squash, sweet potato, and leafy greens
- zinc: eggs, Brazil nuts, pumpkin seeds, pecans, and ginger
- vitamin C: lemons, limes, oranges, Brussels sprouts, and leafy greens
- B vitamins: leafy greens, whole grains, lentils, and bell peppers
- vitamin D: eggs, butter, salmon, mushrooms, and leafy greens

STRENGTHENING AND REBUILDING FOODS

You can become weak and depleted from treatments or from cancer itself. Now, after treatment, is the time to rebuild your strength. Not only will this help repair muscle tissue and nutrient stores, but it will also help increase your energy. Fat and protein are the ingredients to do this. They help the body form hormones, enzymes, and hair, as well as aid in tissue repair to speed up healing time. Eat clean sources of protein, like chicken, turkey, nuts, seeds, beans, and eggs. Add in nourishing oils, such as extra-virgin olive oil, coconut oil, and flax oil.

POST-TREATMENT MENU PLAN

	DAY 1	DAY 2	DAY 3	DAY 4	DAY 5
Breakfast	Silver Dollar Vanilla Pancakes* (page 104)	Classic Granola* (page 98)	Dulse, Egg, and Avocado Special (page 103)	Classic Granola* (page 98)	Dulse, Egg, and Avocado Special (page 103)
Juice/ Smoothie/Elixir	Deep Green and Clean juice (page 85)	Cashew Maca smoothie (page 78)	Hydrating Ginger Lemonade (page 88)	Starter Green smoothie (page 74)	Olympic Gold Milk (page 90)
Lunch	Simple Sushi Bowl (page 164)	Coconut Chicken Fingers* (page 152) + Tamari Roasted Brussels Sprouts (page 180)	Mushroom Walnut "Meatballs"*** (page 159) + Garlic Rapini with Sundried Tomatoes (page 194)	Easy Falafels* (page 168) + Quinoa Tabouli (page 185)	Sweet Potato and Mustard Turkey Burgers* (page 141) + Toasted Sesame Arame and Carrot Kale Sauté (page 178)
Snack	Masala Roasted Chickpeas* (page 216)	Rosemary Currant Hazelnut Crackers* (page 204)	Masala Roasted Chickpeas* (page 216)	Rosemary Currant Hazelnut Crackers* (page 204)	Zesty Blueberry Granola Bars* (page 209)
Dinner	Coconut Chicken Fingers* (page 152) + Tamari Roasted Brussels Sprouts (page 180)	Mushroom Walnut "Meatballs"*** (page 159) + Garlic Rapini with Sundried Tomatoes (page 194)	Easy Falafels* (page 168) + Quinoa Tabouli* (page 185)	Sweet Potato and Mustard Turkey Burgers* (page 141) + Toasted Sesame Arame and Carrot Kale Sauté (page 178)	Healing Miso Soup (page 121) + Rainbow Wraps (page 161)
Dessert	Chocolate Tahini Cookies* (page 226)	Baked Apple Berry Crumble* (page 235)	Chocolate Tahini Cookies* (page 226)	Baked Apple Berry Crumble* (page 235)	Chickpea Chocolate Chip Blondies* (page 238)

* These recipes make several portions, so it's a good idea to make these items in advance and then use them for multiple meals.

** We recommend preparing these recipes in advance, before your treatment. Make large batches of soups and stews and then freeze them so it's easy to defrost and reheat them when you aren't feeling well.

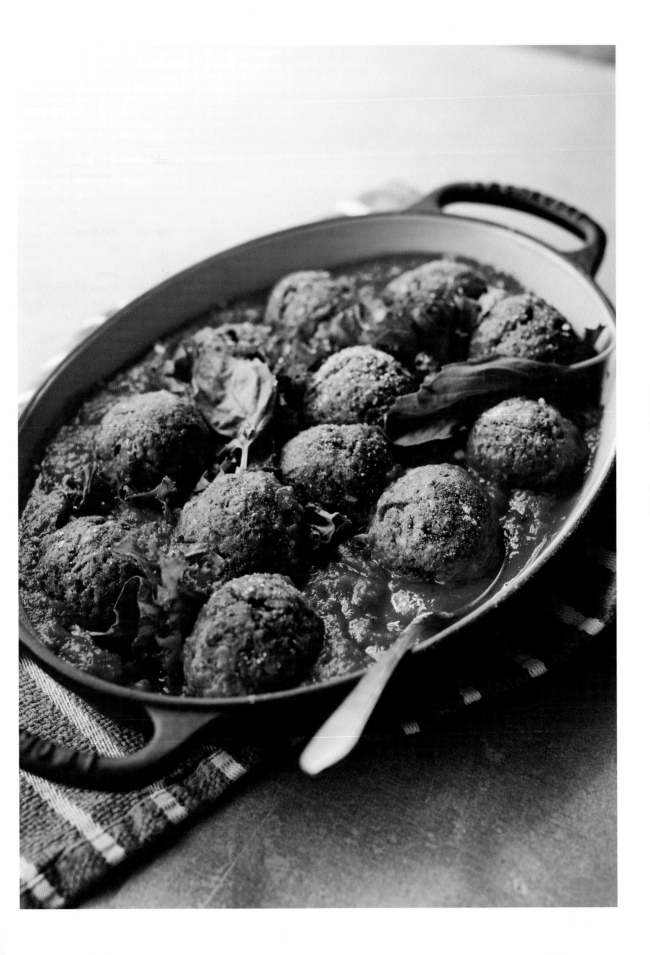

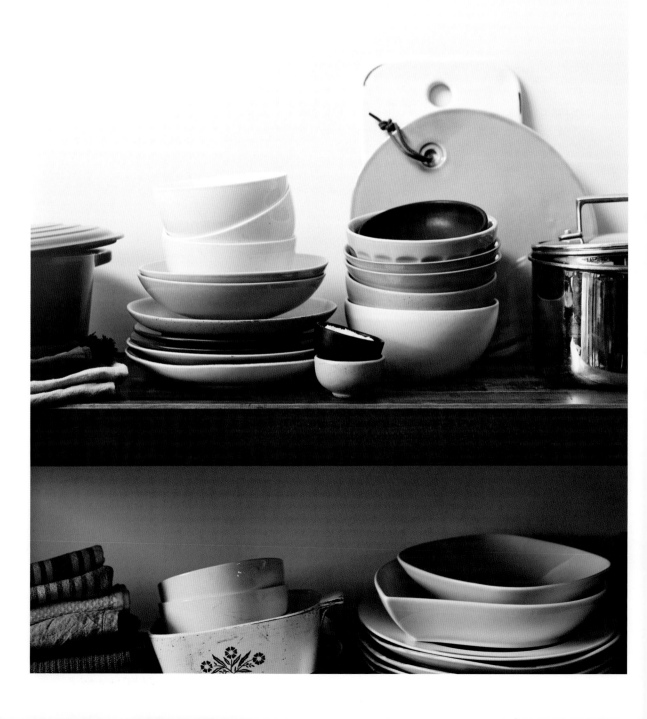

CHAPTER FIVE

Preparing the Kitchen

Before you begin making the recipes, we want to make sure your kitchen is set up with the cooking equipment you need and that you know how to buy the healthiest ingredients. Overhauling your kitchen may not be your first priority as you're preparing for treatment, so we're going to keep it all straightforward and simple. We aren't expecting you to go out and buy a whole new set of cookware or a fancy, expensive blender, but we will make some suggestions on the best items to have in your kitchen. We're going to discuss how to buy organics on a budget, how to buy ingredients wisely, and what cookware you should toss from your kitchen immediately. All of this is vital to set you up for success and make sure you are able to cook the recipes efficiently and with the best and safest ingredients.

BUYING PRODUCE AND ORGANICS ON A BUDGET

While we advocate for purchasing and eating organic produce, we know that it can be quite expensive and sometimes difficult to find every item in the organic section of your grocery store.

Organic produce doesn't use pesticides or chemical insecticides and herbicides, which have been shown to be toxic and carcinogenic. It also is grown in a more nutrient-dense soil, making the food itself more nutritious. Farmers' markets and grocery delivery services are good options for getting organic produce. The latter may be slightly pricier, but the convenience may be worth it for you. However, if organic is not an option, it is better to eat conventional produce than no produce at all.

ORGANIC VERSUS NONORGANIC

If you want to eat organic but are on a budget, here is a solution for you: the Environmental Working Group releases information about which produce items are contaminated with the worst pesticides. This is known as the Dirty Dozen list. When buying produce on a budget, spend your dollars on buying these items organic. The Clean Fifteen is a list of conventional produce that has a lower toxic load of pesticides, meaning these items do not need to be organic for you to eat them. If you are shopping strategically, or have a budget, keep in mind this list of the best conventional produce items to buy. The Environmental Working Group updates these lists each year, so be sure to check its website for changes.

DIRTY DOZEN

In order of "dirtiest" to "dirty," that is, with the most pesticide residues to the least, this is the Dirty Dozen:

Strawberries

Spinach

Nectarines

Apples

Grapes

Peaches

Cherries

Pears

Tomatoes

Celery

Potatoes

Sweet bell peppers

CLEAN FIFTEEN

In order of "cleanest" to least "clean," that is, from the least pesticide residues to the most, these are the Clean Fifteen:

Avocados

Sweet corn

Pineapples

Cabbages

Onions

Frozen sweet peas

Papayas

Asparagus

Mangos

Eggplants

Honeydew melons

Kiwis

Cantaloupes

Cauliflower

Broccoli

Washing and rubbing produce removes pesticides more effectively than just rinsing produce in water alone. If organic isn't an option for you or you need to wash your produce really well because your immune system is low, keep reading.

There are some produce wash products available that advertise their powerful ability to remove pesticides. However, studies have found that water does just as good a job. The truth is there is little to no difference in the reduction of pesticides when using a produce vegetable wash in comparison to using tap water. Just be sure to rinse, rub, scrub, and peel the vegetables and fruits that need it before eating.

HOW TO BUY NUTS AND SEEDS

Choose raw nuts or seeds, rather than salted or roasted. Commercially roasted nuts are usually made with cheap, inflammatory oils. If you have the budget, it's best to buy organic nuts and seeds.

When choosing a nut or seed butter, look at the ingredients and make sure there are no added sugars or oils. Opt for raw or dry-roasted versions (dry roasting doesn't use oil).

If possible, you can also look for sprouted nuts and seeds that have then been dried or dehydrated. Sprouting nuts and seeds increases their nutrient levels and also makes them easier to digest.

HOW TO BUY BEANS AND LEGUMES

To increase the digestibility of dried beans and legumes, like chickpeas, black beans, and white beans, we recommend soaking and, if possible, sprouting them. We realize that this can be a difficult feat for some, so we also recommend buying canned beans and legumes for when you need them in a pinch. Look for cans that have BPA-free lining. Our favorite brands, like Eden, contain seaweed, which reduces the unwanted gassy side effects and improves digestibility (don't worry, you can't taste the seaweed). If you have the time and know-how, soaking and sprouting beans is an incredible way to boost the nutrition profile, increase digestibility, and help the body properly absorb minerals that can sometimes be challenging to access.

HOW TO BUY POULTRY AND RED MEAT

We always recommend purchasing organic and grass-fed animal products when possible. We know this can be expensive, so if you can't get organic animal products, then hormone- and antibiotic-free is the next best option. Animal products are much higher in fat than vegetables, and toxins, hormones, and antibiotics accumulate in fat cells. This means that animal products inherently will have more of these toxins in higher quantities than vegetables because they are fattier.

When it comes to red meat, grass-fed or pasture-raised meat is the best choice. Pasture-raised animals have been raised living outdoors in a pasture or a field. Check for a "100 percent grass-fed" label when buying meat to make sure the animals were actually fed grass and not a combination of grains and grass; their nutritional profile is much healthier for humans to eat.

Our recipes do not contain red meat because of its link with inflammation. However, we do not discourage eating high-quality red meat if that is what your body needs to thrive.

HOW TO BUY FISH AND SEAFOOD

Opt for omega-3-rich fish such as salmon, halibut, anchovies, cod, trout, and sardines. Ideally, you want to buy wild fish or sustainably farmed fish. Most grocery stores or fishmongers will have certifications on their fish noting if they are Marine Stewardship Council, Aqua Stewardship Council, or Seachoice. These certifications indicate whether the fish were sustainably raised or sustainably caught. These are known to contain the least amount of chemical contaminants and be the most environmentally friendly.

HOW TO BUY EGGS

We recommend choosing pasture-raised or organic eggs when possible because they come from chickens living in healthy environments and are not given growth hormones and antibiotics; this makes them more nutritious than eggs from chickens raised on industrial farms.

A FEW HANDY KITCHEN ITEMS WE RECOMMEND

While your kitchen is most likely already equipped with all the tools you need to make our recipes, there are a few items we highly recommend investing in if they're missing from your space.

- A food processor will make your life so much easier and allow you to chop, blend, mix, shred, and mash in a snap.
- A good blender is necessary for making smoothies and blending soups.
- A meat thermometer will ensure that all animal proteins are properly and safely cooked.
- Opt for stainless steel, cast iron, and enameled cast iron (like Le Creuset). Toss unsafe cookware like aluminum and Teflon pans.
- We like to use glass containers and jars to store leftovers in instead of plastic Tupperware, to avoid chemical exposure.

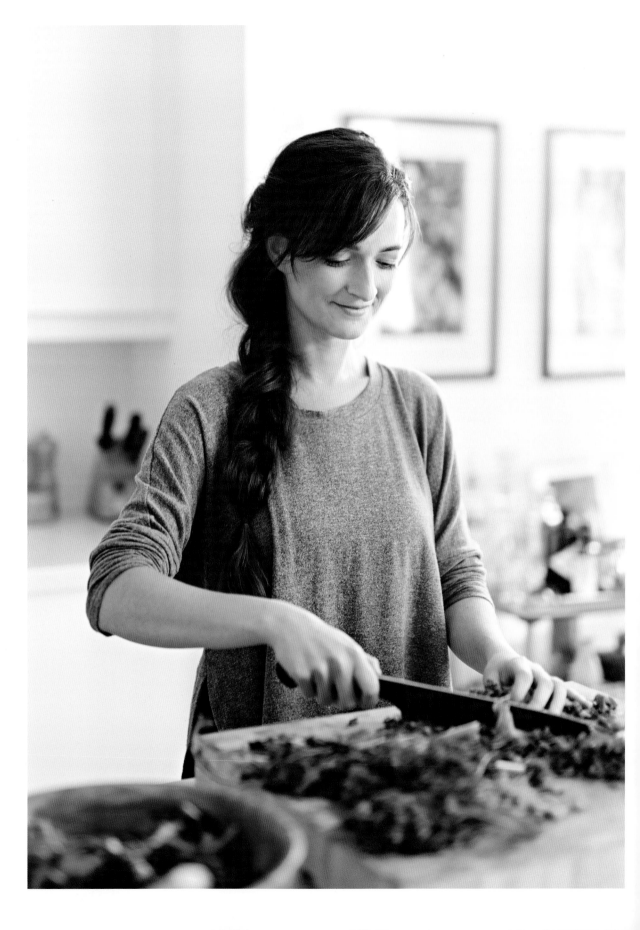

The Recipes

Welcome to the recipes! Flip through the pages and see what inspires you. Because digestion actually begins with your eyes, we recommend that you look at the photographs to help stimulate your appetite and spark your interest for what to make.

We've categorized the recipes by meal type: smoothies, juices and elixirs, breakfasts, soups, omnivore mains, vegetarian mains, sides, snacks, desserts, sauces, marinades, and dressings. If you have trouble swallowing or are experiencing dry mouth or taste changes, we recommend turning to liquid recipes in the soups, smoothies, and juices and elixirs sections. If you feel nauseated, the chapter on snacks offers easy-to-eat, soothing light bites. If your appetite is strong, start with our mains and sides recipes.

We've also included graphic icons with every recipe to guide you on which symptoms our recipes aim to ease.

Our recipes are specifically designed to nourish and support your body during this time. And every dish tastes delicious too. We hope that you will love these recipes as much as we do and find comfort in them when you need it most.

ICONS

≋ eases nausea

Ⓓ helps stop diarrhea

🫃 improves digestion and reduces constipation

💧 stimulates saliva production and helps combat dry mouth and difficulty swallowing

✳ enhances flavors for lost or altered taste buds

👄 eases a sore mouth

⚡ energizes and helps combat fatigue

⚖ encourages healthy weight maintenance

↑ uplifts mood

🍽 stimulates appetite

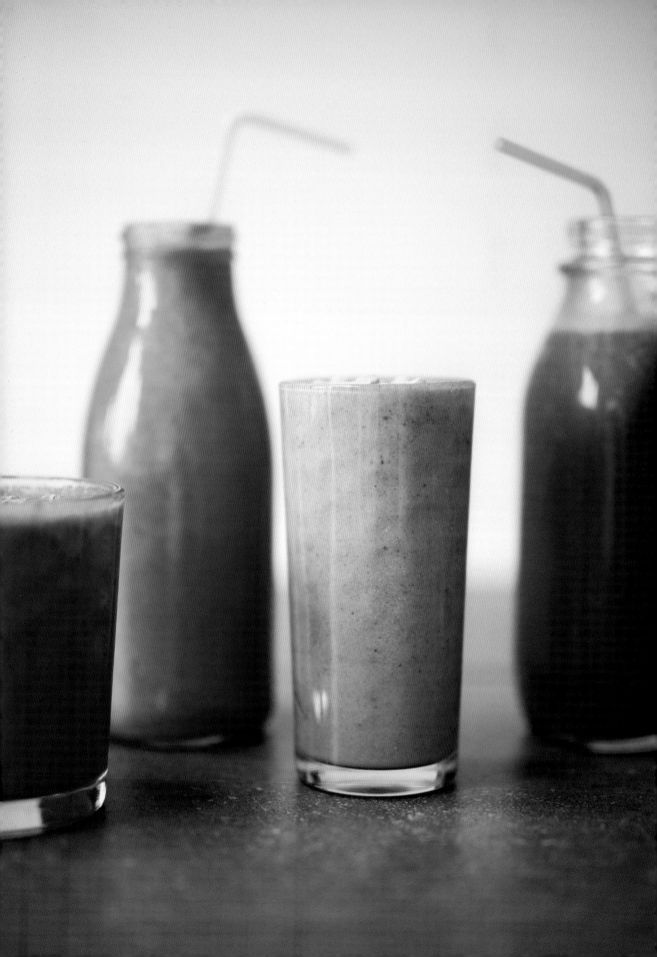

SMOOTHIES

Smoothies are one of the most important, easy-to-digest and easy-to-eat beverages that you can include in your diet right now because your body will quickly absorb the nutrients. Our smoothies incorporate healthy proteins, fats and complex carbs in addition to fresh fruits and vegetables, ensuring that you get all the vital nutrients you need, even if you don't have an appetite.

Our Best Smoothie Tips

1. MAKE EVERY SMOOTHIE THIS WAY

If you're using a high-powered blender, like a Blendtec or Vitamix, the order in which you add your ingredients doesn't really matter. If you don't have one of those, start with the liquid, then add the toughest ingredients (like kale, collards, and beets), and blend until everything is pureed. Now add the rest of your ingredients and blend until a smooth consistency forms.

2. THROW IN EXTRA BOOSTS TO AMP UP YOUR SMOOTHIE

Many of our smoothie recipes have optional add-on superfoods to boost nutrition. Our favorites are listed in the table below.

3. PACK LEFTOVER SMOOTHIE LIKE A PRO (BUT DRINK IT QUICKLY)

If you are using a smoothie as a meal replacement, then you'll probably drink all of it. But if you only want a snack or have a small appetite, then you could always cut the smoothie recipe in half. Store any leftover smoothie in the fridge in an airtight jar; you can drink it up to twenty-four hours after it's been blended.

4. SMOOTHIE PACKS MAKE SMOOTHIES QUICK AND SIMPLE

It's easy to save yourself time and effort by making smoothie packs. Chop all the fresh produce and measure out the dry ingredients for a smoothie in advance, and store them in a ziplock bag or container in the freezer. When you're ready to make a smoothie, simply empty the frozen pack into the blender and add the liquid ingredients. We find that sometimes you need to add a little extra liquid to your blender when the ingredients are frozen to get that smooth consistency.

EXTRA BOOST INGREDIENT	AMOUNT TO USE	HEALTH BENEFIT
Chaga Mushroom Powder	1 tsp	Can kill cancer cells without damaging healthy ones; stimulates the immune system.
Green Powder (Spirulina or Chlorella)	½ tsp	Supports detoxification of chemicals and toxins.
Maca Powder	1 tsp	Increases energy and supports hormonal balance.
Wheatgrass in Frozen Cubes*	1–2 cubes	Has anticancer properties. May work synergistically with chemotherapy. *You can find these in the freezer section of the grocery store.
Slippery Elm Powder	1 tsp	Soothing for sore or irritated throat and mouth.
Raw Cacao Powder	1–2 Tbsp	Flavanols in cacao have anticancer properties.
Probiotics	1 capsule (remove from the capsule)	Important for proper digestion and strengthening the immune system.
Flax Oil	2–3 tsp	Helps reduce inflammation to reduce cancer growth.

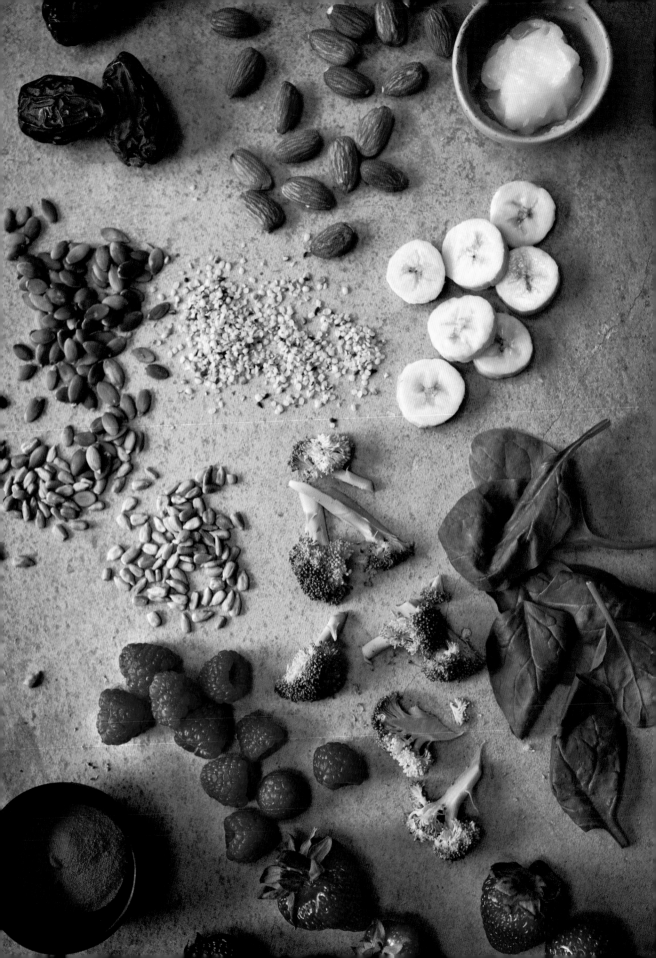

MAKES 1 LARGE SERVING
OR 2 SMALL SERVINGS

———————

1¾ cups unsweetened dairy-
free milk

½ cup frozen cauliflower
(about 5 florets)

½ cup frozen or fresh blueberries

½ cup frozen or fresh
raspberries

¼ cup baby spinach

2 Tbsp hemp seeds

1 Tbsp almond butter (or nut or
seed butter of choice)

1 Tbsp vegan protein powder

1 medjool date, pitted

Restore

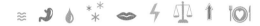

Restore is our Living Kitchen–healthified, upgraded version of commercial protein drinks. Ours isn't filled with cheap sweeteners, refined sugar, dyes, and emulsifiers. Our ingredients may look a little "out there" at first glance, but trust us that this smoothie delivers on both taste and nutrition.

MAKES 1 LARGE SERVING
OR 2 SMALL SERVINGS

———————

1½ cups unsweetened dairy-
free milk

1 cup kale or spinach

1 banana, peeled

2 Tbsp hemp seeds

1 Tbsp almond butter (or other
nut or seed butter)

Extra Boosts:

1 frozen cube wheatgrass

½ tsp spirulina

1 Tbsp vegan protein powder

1–2 medjool dates, pitted

The Starter Green

This smoothie is a simple and tasty way to get anticancer greens into your diet and support your healthy cells. This is a great place to start if you're new to green smoothies. Years ago, when I first entered the nutrition field and green smoothies were about to hit their popularity peak, this smoothie was my go-to. Years later, it's still part of my morning repertoire, and even my young son gobbles it up. When a kid will drink it, you know it really has the stamp of approval. **TG**

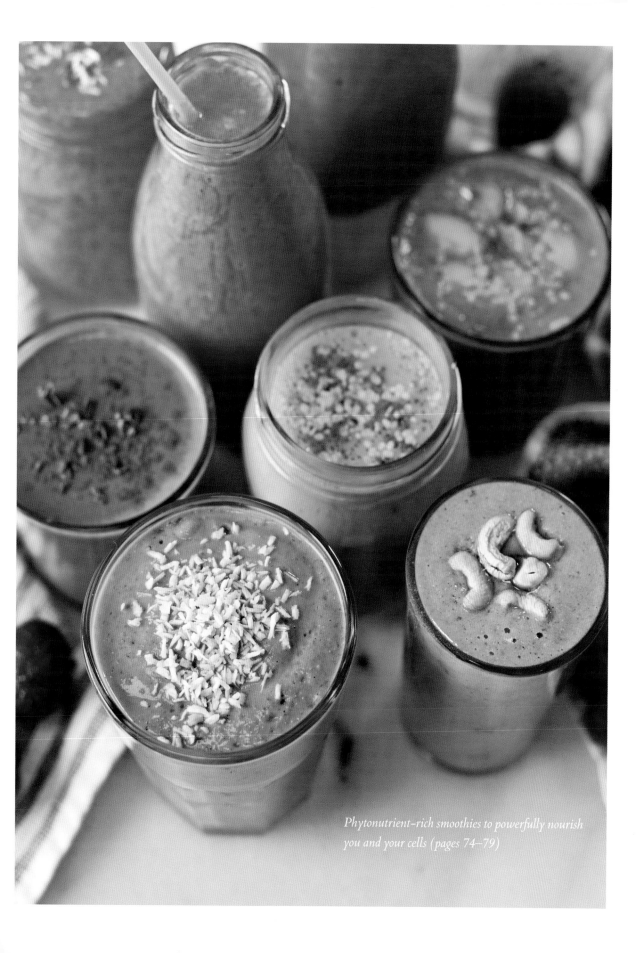

Phytonutrient–rich smoothies to powerfully nourish you and your cells (pages 74–79)

---

1 cup unsweetened dairy-free
    milk

½ cup full-fat coconut milk

½ cup baby spinach

¼ avocado, peeled

3 medjool dates, pitted

2 Tbsp raw cacao powder

2 Tbsp raw cashews

1 heaping Tbsp almond butter
    (or nut or seed butter of
    choice)

¼ tsp cinnamon

Extra Boosts:

1 tsp chaga mushroom powder

1 frozen cube wheatgrass

1 tsp maca powder

1 tsp slippery elm powder

Chocolate Almond

To all the chocoholics out there: this one is for you. This smoothie is a great starter beverage if you're new to the smoothie game. It tastes like you're drinking a delicious chocolate milkshake, not a hearty, nutritious drink filled with antioxidants, healthy fat, protein, and fiber. If you need a chocolate fix in your life, make this one immediately. Bonus: it'll fuel you during treatment days too.

NUTRITION NOTE Chaga mushroom powder is an optional add-on but we highly recommend you use it. Chaga helps modulate the immune system, meaning it can suppress or stimulate your immune system based on what your body needs.

MAKES 1 LARGE SERVING
OR 2 SMALL SERVINGS

———————

½ cup unsweetened dairy-free
    milk

½ cup unsweetened coconut
    water

2 Tbsp coarsely chopped beet
    (raw or cooked)

10 small or 5 large strawberries,
    chopped

½ banana, peeled

⅓ cup orange segments

½ tsp minced peeled ginger
    root

½ tsp turmeric

Pinch of pepper

Superfood Beet

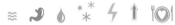

We absolutely adore this smoothie's bright pink color, courtesy of the phytonutrients in the beets and strawberries. Fruit
gives the smoothie a sweet flavor, and you'll be happily surprised by how the citrus calms the earthiness of the beets—so
much so that you can barely taste them. Ginger gives this a little
extra spicy kick, which will help altered taste buds and nausea.

NUTRITION NOTE The
turmeric in this smoothie provides potent anti-inflammatory
properties, and the pinch of
pepper helps increase the
absorbability of the turmeric.

MAKES 1 LARGE SERVING
OR 2 SMALL SERVINGS

———————

1½ cups unsweetened dairy-
    free milk

1 cup fresh or frozen mango

½ banana, peeled

2 Tbsp hemp seeds

1 Tbsp virgin coconut oil

1 Tbsp almond butter

1 tsp turmeric

½ tsp minced peeled ginger
    root

Pinch of pepper

Extra Boost:
1 Tbsp vegan protein powder

Golden Ginger

Over the years, we've tried making smoothies with kale,
spirulina, nuts, and other nourishing ingredients that,
unfortunately, don't always make the most appetizing-looking
smoothie. But this smoothie wins the day with a bright,
uplifting color (thanks to the turmeric, which studies show
can prevent cancer cells from growing). We feel happier just
looking at it. And the tropical flavors of mango and banana are
all you'll taste; you won't even know the turmeric is there.

Greena Colada

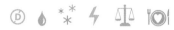

MAKES 1 LARGE SERVING
OR 2 SMALL SERVINGS

½ cup unsweetened dairy-free
milk

½ cup unsweetened coconut
milk

½ cup baby spinach

½ cup fresh or frozen pineapple
cubes

½ small banana, peeled

¼ small avocado, peeled

2 tsp virgin coconut oil

2 tsp unsweetened shredded
coconut

2 tsp chia seeds

Extra Boosts:
½ tsp slippery elm powder

½ tsp spirulina

1 frozen cube wheatgrass

This is our delicious take on a piña colada, but minus the alcohol and getting caught in the rain. Our Greena Colada tastes so refreshing and tropical, you won't even believe that your cells are being nourished with avocado, spinach, and chia.

NUTRITION NOTE The boatload of coconut in this recipe (full-fat coconut milk, coconut oil, and shredded coconut) is an excellent and easy way to add great fat to your diet. Pineapple helps make this drink easy on the stomach, as it naturally contains bromelain, a digestive enzyme.

Cashew Maca

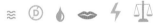

MAKES 1 LARGE SERVING
OR 2 SMALL SERVINGS

---

1 cup unsweetened dairy-free
milk

½ cup full-fat coconut milk

1 banana, peeled

¼ cup raw cashews

2 medjool dates, pitted

1 Tbsp virgin coconut oil

1 tsp maca powder

¼ tsp cinnamon

⅛ tsp nutmeg or cardamom

This dreamy, creamy smoothie is sweetly spiced and a true pleasure to drink. Its silky texture is gentle and smooth. While this smoothie may taste like dessert, it actually does so much more for you—like boost your mood, energy, and memory.

Extra Boosts:
1 Tbsp chia seeds

1 tsp chaga mushroom powder

½ tsp pure vanilla extract

————

1½ cups unsweetened dairy-
free milk

1 cup baby spinach

1 cup fresh or frozen
strawberries, hulled

½ cup fresh or frozen
blueberries

½ cup fresh or frozen
raspberries

1 Tbsp virgin coconut oil

1 Tbsp nut or seed butter of
choice

1 Tbsp hemp seeds

Extra Boosts:

1 Tbsp vegan protein powder

1 tsp slippery elm powder

½ tsp spirulina

1 frozen cube wheatgrass

NUTRITION NOTE Berries
have a lot of things going for
them: deep, rich, gorgeous colors
courtesy of phytonutrients that
reduce inflammation and provide
antioxidant support, and querce-
tin, a nutrient that may inhibit
tumor growth.

Blended Berry

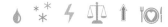

When we think of the flavors of a classic smoothie, without
a doubt, we always think of berries. Berries naturally taste
sweet and always remind us of summer, even if we drink this
smoothie in the middle of winter. We love combining sweet
strawberries with tart blueberries and raspberries. To take
it up a notch, we've added greens, a powerhouse anticancer
ingredient, but you won't taste them!

We've kept this smoothie low glycemic by making it without banana or
dates. If it's not sweet enough for you, add a few drops of stevia to make
it a low-sugar smoothie.

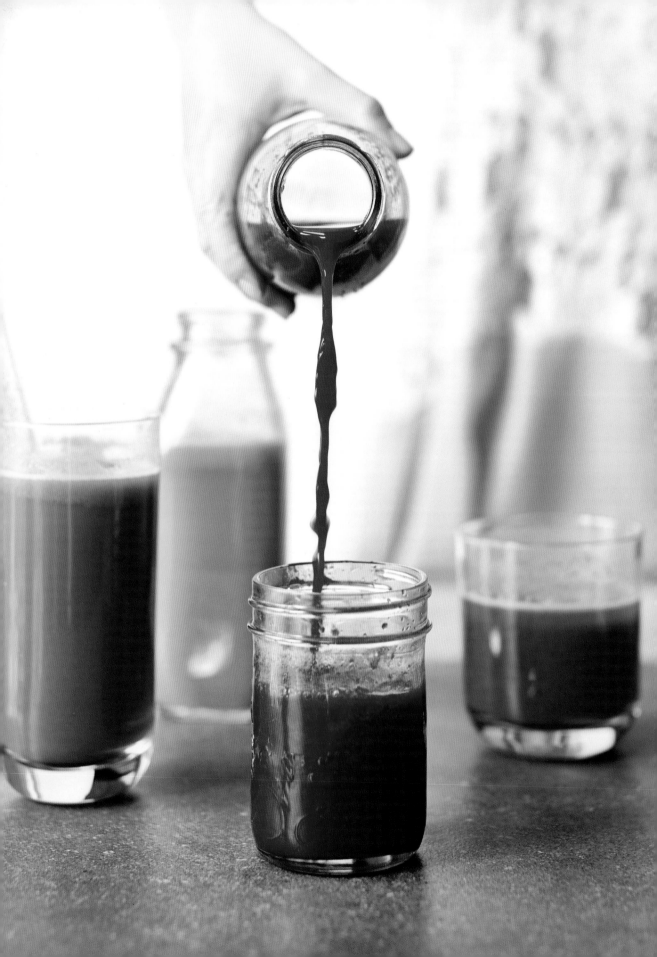

JUICES AND ELIXIRS

Juices are a fast way to supply your body with vitamins, minerals, and phytonutrients that are quick and easy to absorb. The process of juicing removes fiber from the fruits and veggies, so nutrients are delivered to your body immediately. And because juices are raw, all the enzymes in the produce remain intact, which supports your digestion as you drink up. Our elixirs combine a medley of powerhouse ingredients that gently hydrate and energize you while also helping to ease common side effects like nausea, digestive discomfort, and fatigue.

A How-To for All of Our Juices (pages 83–86)

1. USE RAW VEGETABLES AND FRUITS FOR THESE RECIPES.

2. RINSE OFF VEGETABLES AND FRUITS WITH WATER.
You can scrub tough-skinned vegetables such as cucumbers, beets, carrots, and ginger to remove dirt.

3. YOU CAN LEAVE THE SKINS ON ORGANIC VEGETABLES, SUCH AS CARROTS, BEETS, AND APPLES.
We usually take the tough peel off fruits like lemons and oranges, since they can be hard on your juicer. Try to keep the white part (the pith) on lemons and oranges because it is rich in vitamin C.

4. IF YOU'RE USING CONVENTIONAL NONORGANIC PRODUCE, IT IS BEST TO REMOVE THE SKINS AND PEELS TO AVOID PESTICIDES.

5. CUT VEGETABLES AND FRUITS INTO SMALL PIECES THAT WILL FIT THROUGH YOUR JUICER TUBE.

6. FEED THE INGREDIENTS THROUGH YOUR JUICER ONE BY ONE TO AVOID JAMMING IT.

7. IT'S BEST TO DRINK YOUR JUICE IMMEDIATELY AFTER PREPARATION TO GET ALL THE ACTIVE VITAMINS AND ANTIOXIDANTS.
But if you can't drink it right away, you can store the juice in an airtight jar in the refrigerator for 24–48 hours.

MAKES 1 LARGE SERVING
OR 2 SMALLER SERVINGS

---

4 kale leaves and stems

1 cucumber

1 cup cubed fresh pineapple,
   skin removed

1 inch ginger root

5 fresh mint leaves and stems
   (you can add more if you
   love mint or omit if you don't
   like it)

Kickstarter Kale

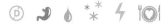

Are you a juicing newbie? This is a great "kickstarter" juice for all you beginners out there. Some green juices can be really intense, but this one has a gentler and sweeter flavor, thanks to pineapple and mint. Pineapple is also a powerful digestive aid—you can credit the enzyme bromelain for that. So, if your stomach needs some love, this juice is one to drink up!

MAKES 1 LARGE SERVING
OR 2 SMALLER SERVINGS

---

2 beets

3 ribs celery

1 medium carrot

½ peeled orange

½ peeled lemon

1 inch ginger root

Citrus Beet

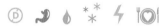

Our Citrus Beet juice has a bright, rich, beautiful reddish-purple color that's not only nice to look at but is also responsible for providing liver and detoxification support. If green juices aren't your thing, this beet juice is where it's at. The taste is refreshingly citrusy, earthy, and mildly zippy.

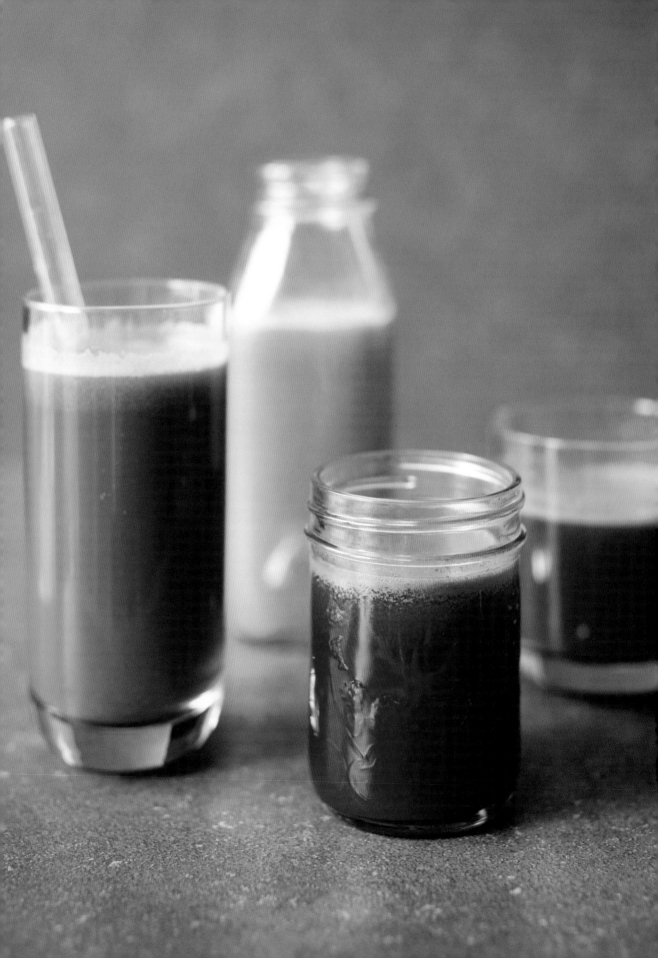

---

4 ribs celery

1 large or 2 small kale leaves and stems

½ medium cucumber

½ green apple

½ peeled lemon

1½ inches ginger root

Deep Green and Clean

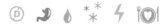

Are you ready for some deep, green cleaning? This power-house juice is our go-to recommendation for anyone feeling sick or fatigued from treatment, because it truly energizes the body and supplies quick nutrients. It also works to detoxify heavy metals and radiation from your body. The ginger gives this juice a mildly spicy flavor that can also relieve nausea.

1½ cups broccoli florets and stem

2 ribs celery

½ medium cucumber

1 pear

½ peeled lemon

NUTRITION NOTE Phyto-nutrients found within cucumbers may actually block signaling pathways for cancer cells.

Broccoli Pear

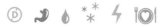

Broccoli in juice? Yes, it sounds weird. No, we're not crazy. Eating a bowl of broccoli can be challenging for many who are going through treatment, so one way to get the incredible benefits of this superfood vegetable is to juice it! Juicing broccoli will help you get its detoxification and anticancer properties. And the pear and lemon both help to balance the bitter flavor of broccoli, making this a surprisingly refreshing juice.

————————

4 ribs celery

½ medium cucumber

½ peeled lemon

½ peeled orange

1 inch ginger root

1 inch fresh turmeric root

½ garlic clove

NUTRITION NOTE These ingredients reduce inflammation and possess antibacterial, anti-microbial, and antiviral properties while stimulating your body's detoxification system to remove cancerous chemicals and toxins.

Immunity Zip

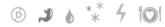

When your immune system needs some serious support, it's time to gulp our Immunity Zip juice.

Lemon, ginger, turmeric, garlic, and orange are the major players in the immunity game, and though you may be wary of garlic in a juice, you'll find this juice tastes like orange and lemon with a nice kick of ginger.

If you don't have fresh turmeric root, you can stir 1 teaspoon of turmeric powder into the juice. If you are sensitive to raw garlic, you can omit it, or start out with using even less than half a clove.

2 cups water or unsweetened
   coconut water

2 Tbsp fresh lemon juice

2 tsp pure maple syrup

⅛ tsp sea salt

NUTRITION NOTE Sea salt
naturally contains electrolytes,
and adding a pinch of it to a glass
of water is one of the easiest
ways to replace lost electrolytes.
Maple syrup provides carbohydrates to give your cells some
energy and helps balance out
the salt.

Energizing Electrolyte Drink

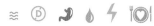

We always hear about how important it is to drink water and
stay hydrated. But sometimes plain water just isn't enough
when you're in the middle of cancer treatment. If you've lost
fluids, it's extremely important to replace electrolytes like
magnesium, potassium, calcium, and sodium, because they're
all essential in regulating your cellular function in every part
of your body. Without them your cells can't hold onto water
and actually rehydrate. Although you can detect the taste of
sea salt in this drink, you'll find it tastes more of lemon and is
subtly sweet from the maple syrup. You can make this recipe
instead of buying electrolyte drinks that are full of chemicals
and artificial ingredients.

1. Pour the water, lemon juice, maple syrup, and salt into
   a mason jar or water bottle.
2. Screw the lid on and shake to mix everything together.
3. Drink right away or store in the refrigerator for up to
   3 days.

If you want to boost the electrolyte power, use coconut water instead of
plain water. If it tastes too salty for you, you can add ½ cup of orange or
apple juice to this recipe.

3 cups water

⅓ cup fresh lemon juice

1 inch ginger root, peeled and chopped

8 drops of liquid stevia (or more if you like it sweeter)

NUTRITION NOTE You'll get vitamin C from the lemon and antinausea benefits and immune support from the ginger.

Hydrating Ginger Lemonade

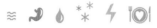

As a kid I'd beg my mom to buy pink lemonade. I thought it looked so delicious, and on hot summer days I'd dream about it, but my mom knew better then to buy artificially colored drinks that would just give my sister and me a sugar high. Fast-forward to now, and there's nothing I love more on a hot day than sipping homemade, sugar-free lemonade with ginger. We developed this recipe many years ago for one of our clients who loves lemonade but wanted to avoid eating sugar during cancer therapy, and then we ended up falling in love with this refreshing combo of sweet and sour. Even if you're wary of stevia, give this recipe a try. It'll help keep you hydrated during treatment. **SG**

1. Place all the ingredients except the stevia in a blender and blitz until smooth. The ginger should be completely blended in.
2. Stir in the stevia to your taste preference.
3. Enjoy over ice right away. You can store this in a glass jar in the fridge for up to 3 days and pour it over ice when you're ready to drink.

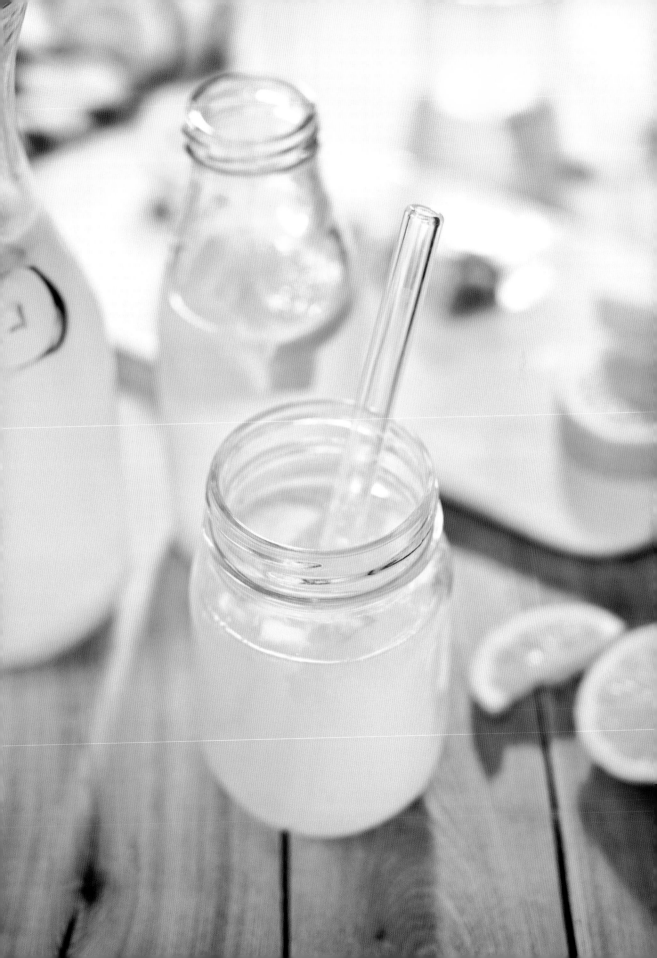

1½ cups unsweetened dairy-
free milk

1 tsp turmeric

¼ tsp cinnamon

¼ tsp ground ginger

Pinch of black pepper

6 drops of liquid stevia (or
more if you like it sweeter)

Olympic Gold Milk

I've always been a huge chai latte fan—I love the comforting, rich spices mixed with creamy milk in a chai latte, but the coffee shop versions are often loaded with sugar. So we came up with something that's even better: it's creamy like a chai latte but with immune-strengthening turmeric and a beautiful golden color. Cinnamon and ginger add warmth and balance out the bitter taste of turmeric, and you can make it completely sugar-free. Enjoy this with breakfast or later in the day as a treat—it's an easy way to increase your turmeric intake, which has many cancer-fighting properties, like inhibiting cancer cell growth. Credit for the name goes to one of our clients, who loved this drink and drank it religiously as she watched the Olympics. **SG**

1. Add all the ingredients except the stevia to a small pot on the stove.
2. Whisk the spices into the milk until they are dissolved and everything is combined.
3. Heat gently on medium until just below boiling. Pour into a mug, add the stevia to taste, and enjoy.

If you don't like stevia, you can add 1 to 2 tsp honey or coconut sugar to sweeten this instead.

1½ cups unsweetened dairy-free milk

1 tsp matcha powder

1 Tbsp hot water

1 Tbsp virgin coconut oil

6 drops of liquid stevia (or more if you like it sweeter) or 1–2 tsp honey

NUTRITION NOTE Matcha tea is rich in epigallocatechin-3-gallate (EGCG), a compound that researchers have linked with preventing cancer. It's best to buy organic matcha, even if it seems expensive, as you'll want the higher-quality tea to get the most health benefits. And a little bit of matcha goes a long way!

Miracle Matcha Latte

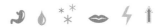

Sipping a hot, frothy cup of tea is a wonderful way to start off the day or to unwind in the afternoon. But we recommend limiting caffeine during treatment. We understand this can be a real challenge if you're a caffeine lover, so we've come up with an alternative for you. Matcha, made from ground green tea leaves, contains some caffeine (but a lot less than coffee), and might just do the trick if you want something with a little kick of energy. Enjoy this vibrantly colored green tea that's naturally sweet and earthy, and that tastes so smooth whisked into dairy-free milk.

1. Add the milk to a small pot on the stove. Heat gently on medium until just below boiling.
2. Meanwhile, whisk the matcha powder with 1 tablespoon of hot water in a mug until there are no clumps and it's a smooth mixture.
3. Once the milk is hot, pour it into the mug with the matcha.
4. Pour the matcha and milk mixture into a blender and add the coconut oil. Blend for 30 seconds, or until the coconut oil is emulsified into the liquid. This will help make the milk frothy.
5. Pour into the mug, add stevia or honey to taste, and enjoy.

You'll need a whisk to blend the matcha powder into the liquid. You can find a matcha tea whisk at any tea shop or on the internet. If you don't have a tea whisk, you can use a regular small whisk.

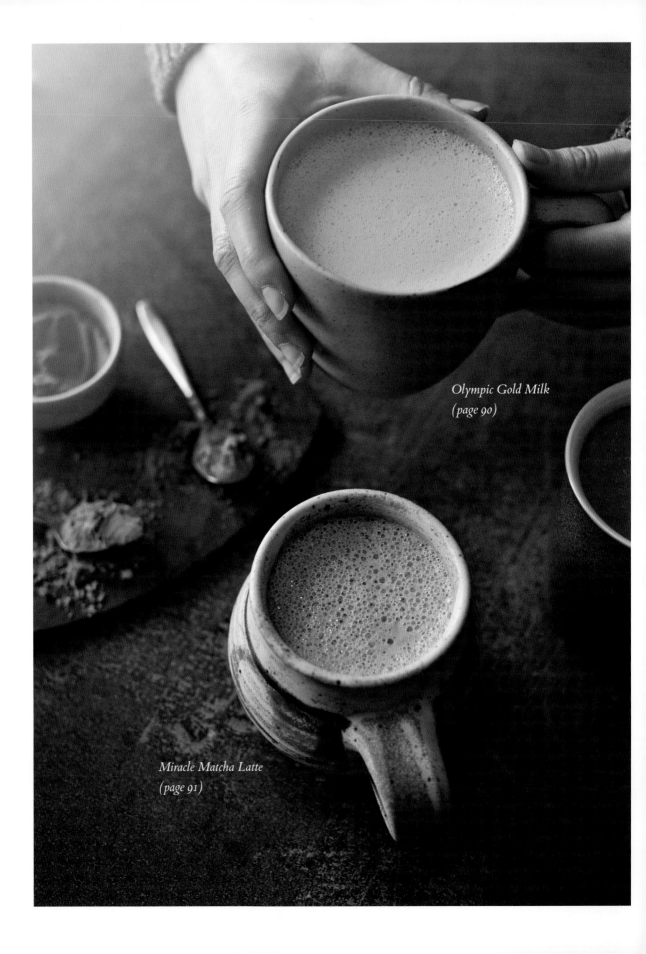

Olympic Gold Milk
(page 90)

Miracle Matcha Latte
(page 91)

4 cups water

3 inches ginger root, peeled and thinly sliced

1 lemon, juiced

6 drops of liquid stevia (or more if you like it sweeter) or 1–2 tsp honey

Fresh Ginger Tea

My grandmother had all the remedies: gargle with salt water if you had a sore throat, sip a cup of chicken soup when you had a cold, and drink ginger lemon tea whenever you felt sick. She was always spot-on with her remedy recommendations. Fresh ginger tea provides incredible immune-supportive and anti-inflammatory benefits, and it's the best tool we have to deal with treatment-related nausea, digestive discomfort, and sore throats. **TG**

1. Add the water and ginger to a small pot over medium heat. Bring the mixture to a boil, cover, and allow it to simmer for 10 minutes.
2. Remove the pot from the heat and pour in the lemon juice and stevia. If you aren't going to drink this tea all in one sitting, you can always reheat it on the stove top later on.
4. This tea can be stored in a glass jar in the fridge for up to 3 days. Reheat just before serving.

If you're not a fan of ginger pieces swimming in your tea as you drink, strain them out before adding the lemon juice and stevia.

1 cup full-fat coconut milk

1 Tbsp raw cacao powder

¼ tsp cinnamon

¼ tsp ground ginger

Pinch of cayenne pepper

6 drops of liquid stevia (or more if you like it sweeter) or 2 tsp maple syrup

Extra Boost:
1 tsp ground chaga mushroom

NUTRITION NOTE Raw cacao is the unprocessed form of chocolate (yes, that means it's healthy chocolate!) that helps boost your mood. If you want more of a classic hot chocolate, just leave out the spices.

Spiced Hot Chocolate

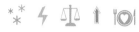

I was living in an unheated apartment in the dead of winter. Desperate for warmth, I decided to whisk up a version of hot chocolate with some random ingredients I had in my pantry. I poured all the ingredients into a pot and accidentally set it on high heat before turning away for a second. Suddenly my hot chocolate was about to bubble over and explode out of the pot. I grabbed the pot just in time, and my drink settled down into a frothy masterpiece. The secret to making this drink divine is to let it get to the point where it's about to spill over—and then catch it just in time. Really. And not only is this drink chocolaty, sweet, and spicy, but it also supports the immune system and eases stomachaches. **TG**

1. Add all the ingredients except for the stevia to a small pot and whisk the spices into the milk. If you are using maple syrup instead of stevia, add that to the pot with the other ingredients.
2. Simmer on low heat until just below the boiling point, when the mixture begins to froth up.
3. Remove from the heat immediately and mix in the stevia to desired sweetness. Enjoy right away.

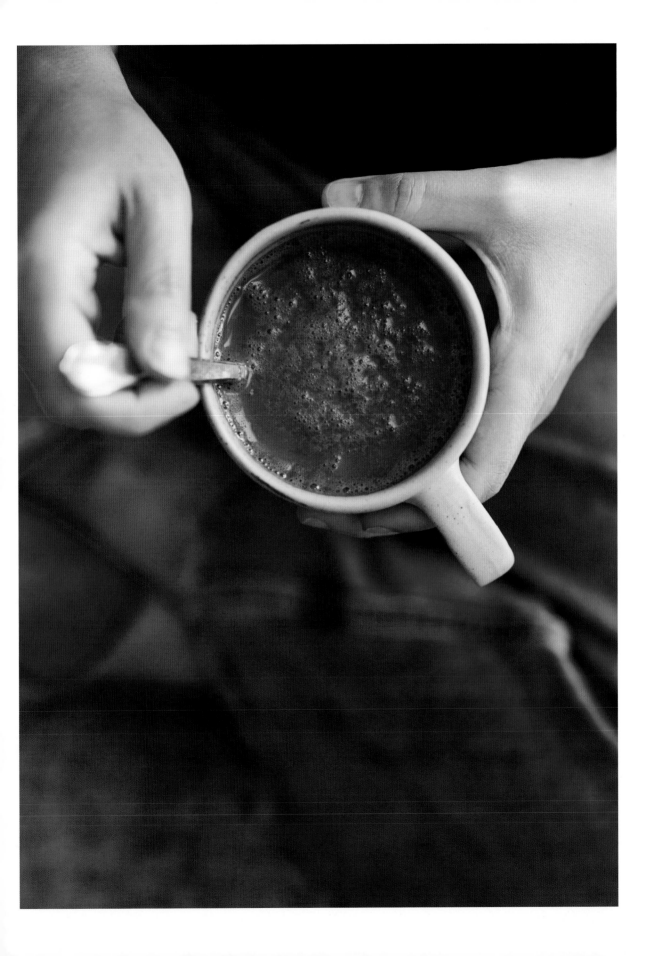

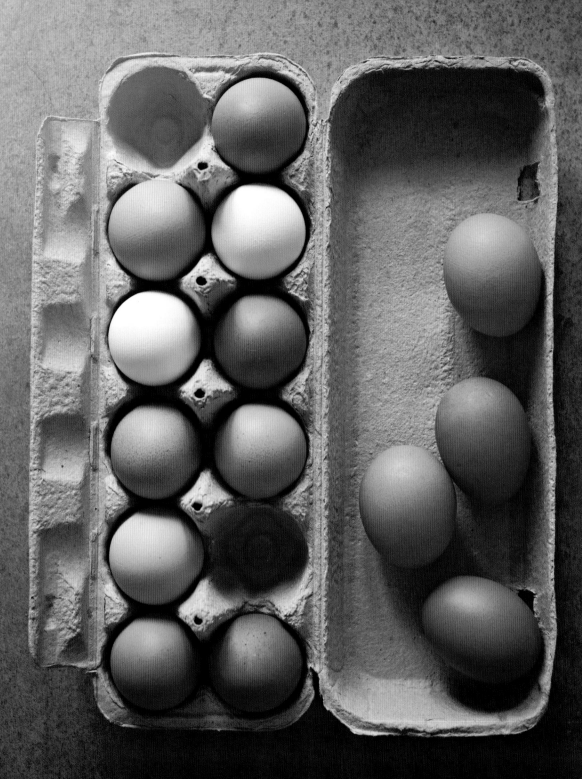

BREAKFASTS

Breakfast is widely known as the most important meal of the day, and for good reason: it's the meal that sets you up and literally fuels your body. During treatment, breakfast may help stimulate your appetite when you don't have one, which in turn may help offset side effects like nausea and fatigue. We've incorporated a good mix of sweet and savory breakfasts here, so you have many tasty options to choose from. These recipes are in the breakfast section, but you can always enjoy them as lunch, dinner, or snacks.

———————

3 cups rolled oats or quick oats

½ cup raw Brazil nuts, coarsely chopped

½ cup raw walnuts

½ cup unsweetened coconut flakes

⅓ cup raw sunflower seeds

⅓ cup raw pumpkin seeds

½ tsp cinnamon

Pinch of sea salt

⅓ cup virgin coconut oil, melted

¼ cup pure maple syrup

½ cup goji berries

½ cup cacao nibs

NUTRITION NOTE The Brazil nuts are an important part of this granola. They are rich in selenium, a protective antioxidant that fights against cancer. Goji berries and cacao nibs add more antioxidants and make this granola delicious.

Classic Granola

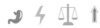

I love the smell of cinnamon, maple syrup, and toasted oats wafting from the oven. It's the smell of homemade granola. Granola was one of the first recipes I made when I started cooking, because it's my all-time favorite breakfast, especially paired with coconut yogurt and fresh fruit. I also love how easy it is to get creative and add different nuts, seeds, and dried fruit to make variations. Plus, it's so much better than sugar-filled store-bought granola, because you decide how much sweetener to add. Not only is our Classic Granola a satisfying breakfast, but it can also double as a snack throughout the day, when you have doctor's appointments or treatment. **SG**

1. Preheat the oven to 350°F and line a baking sheet with parchment paper.
2. In a large bowl, mix together the oats, Brazil nuts, walnuts, coconut flakes, sunflower seeds, pumpkin seeds, cinnamon, and salt.
3. Melt the coconut oil in a small pot on the stove top over medium-low heat until it liquefies. Add the maple syrup. Then, using a spatula, fold the liquid mixture into the dry ingredients.
4. Spread the granola out onto the baking sheet and bake for 25 minutes, or until lightly browned. Stir the granola after 15 minutes.
5. Remove from the oven and mix in the goji berries and cacao nibs.
6. Enjoy the granola served over dairy-free coconut yogurt or with dairy-free milk. It's delicious to add some fresh berries too! Store in a sealed glass jar for up to 2 months.

If you don't eat oats, you can substitute quinoa flakes. And if you can't find goji berries, use other dried fruit, like dried cherries, mulberries, golden berries, or even raisins. Just make sure that the fruit has no added sugar, as it's naturally sweet enough.

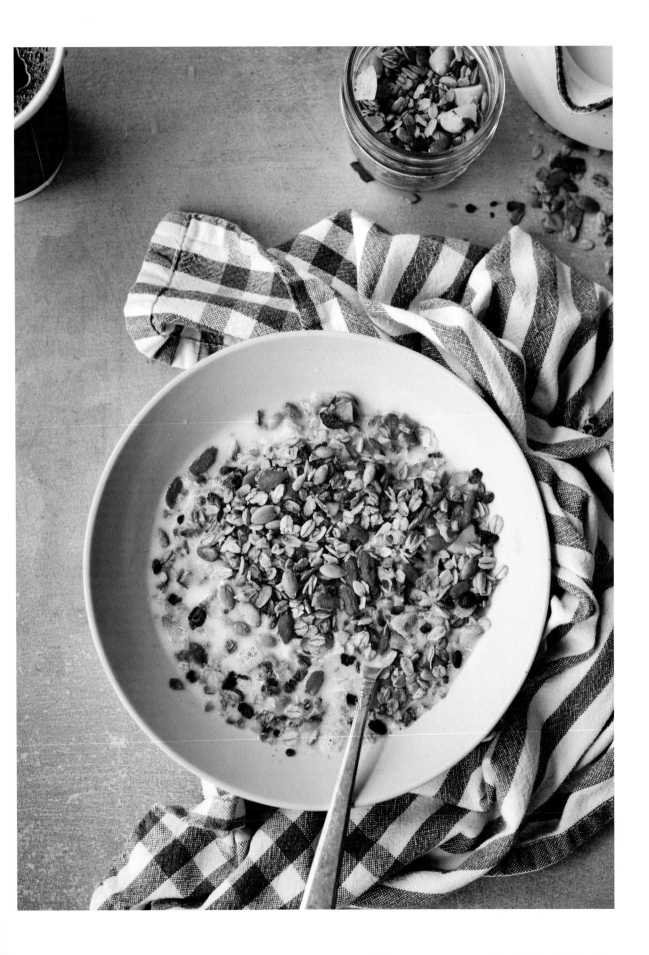

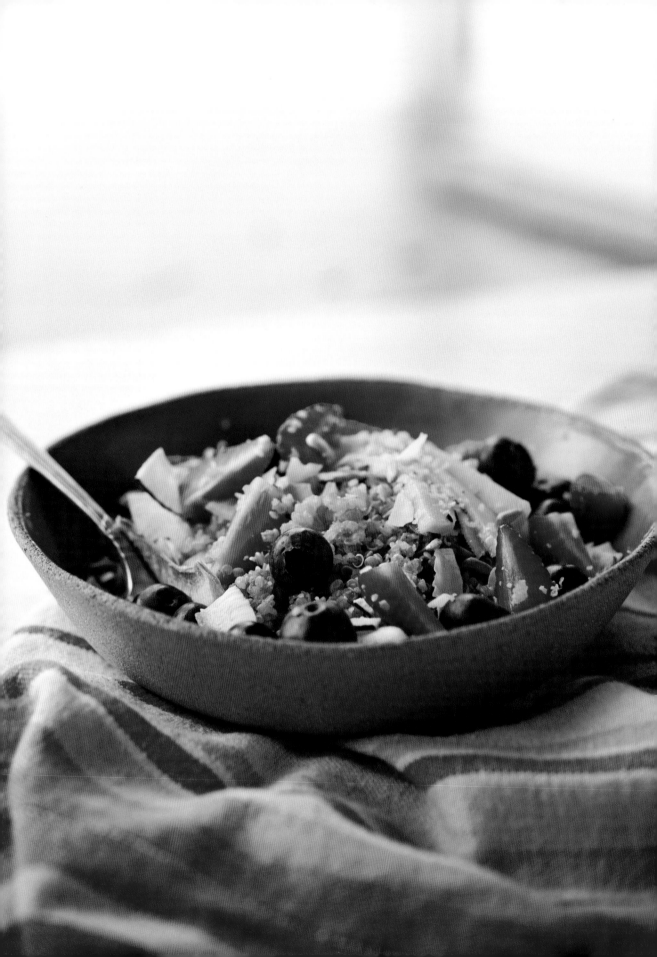

———————

½ cup quinoa

1 cup water

¼ tsp cinnamon

¼ tsp ground ginger

½ tsp turmeric

1 tsp pure maple syrup
(optional; omit if you follow
a sugar-free diet)

1 Tbsp raw sunflower seeds

1 Tbsp raw pumpkin seeds

2 tsp unsweetened shredded
coconut

2 tsp hemp seeds

Large handful of fresh berries
(blueberries, strawberries,
raspberries, or blackberries)

NUTRITION NOTE There are
some powerful spices at work
in this recipe. Turmeric, ginger,
and cinnamon all help prevent
the growth of cancer cells and
inflammation. Ginger is also one
of the best foods for reducing
nausea.

Cinnamon Quinoa Breakfast Bowl

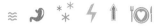

Quinoa isn't just for lunch and dinner. Not only does it provide protein, B vitamins, zinc, and fiber, but it also has a warm flavor that's perfect in the morning—and it's a great gluten-free option, with more nutrients than a piece of toast. If you're craving a sweeter but still healthy and filling breakfast, our Cinnamon Quinoa Breakfast Bowl is the one for you. And it's a fantastic alternative to oatmeal.

1. In a small pot, combine the quinoa and water. Bring it to a boil, reduce to a simmer, cover, and cook on low heat for 15 minutes.
2. Once the quinoa is cooked and fluffy, add the cinnamon, ginger, turmeric, and maple syrup and mix well.
3. Place in a bowl and top with sunflower seeds, pumpkin seeds, coconut, hemp seeds, and berries.

This is the perfect recipe to make in advance to save yourself time in the morning. You can make a batch of quinoa and store it in the fridge, then just warm it up for breakfast.

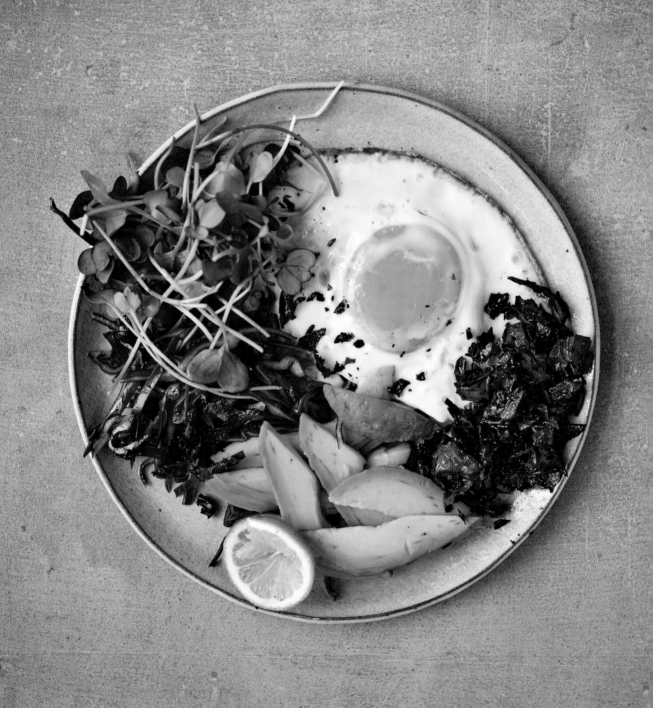

---

2 tsp ghee or extra-virgin
olive oil

2 eggs

⅓ cup dried dulse

¼–½ avocado, sliced into
thin strips

Large handful of sprouts

2–3 Tbsp sauerkraut

NUTRITION NOTE Dulse adds
another level of flavor, but, more
importantly, a rich serving of nutrients like iron, iodine, calcium,
and magnesium—all of which
support the body in removing
toxins. Seaweed also protects
DNA, helping to prevent cancer.
Avocado is a wonderful source
of healthy fat and can help keep
your calorie and fat intake up if
you're dealing with weight loss.

Dulse, Egg, and Avocado Special

I always get so excited when someone tells me they love dulse!
Although I know most people have never heard of this delicious, salty, and crispy-when-sautéed seaweed, I really believe
it's one of the most tasty and interesting foods out there,
especially if you like salty, savory things, as I do. This recipe
came to be when I got tired of eating plain old sunny-side-up
eggs. The sauerkraut is an easy way to support your digestion
and immune system, and dulse is the perfect complement to
eggs, especially when you add avocado. Some even say it's the
best substitute for bacon, but you'll have to try it for yourself
and see! **SG**

1. Heat a wide pan over medium heat. Add the ghee, swirling
   it around to coat the bottom. Carefully crack the eggs into
   the pan. Cook for 2 minutes on one side, until the white
   is opaque. Then flip the eggs over and cook for another
   minute. We're aiming for over-easy eggs, but if you need
   the yolk to be fully cooked, then leave them in the pan for
   another minute, or until the center is solid.

2. Remove the eggs from the pan and transfer to a plate. In
   the same pan, sauté the dulse for 1–2 minutes to crisp it up
   quickly.

3. Place the dulse next to the eggs and add avocado, a handful
   of sprouts, and sauerkraut. Enjoy right away.

You can find dulse at health food stores or online. It usually comes in
2- to 3-inch-long pieces. Break them in half to make cooking easier.

---

2 eggs

1½ cups blanched almond flour

½ cup unsweetened dairy-free milk

1 Tbsp virgin coconut oil, softened + 2–3 tsp coconut oil for frying

2 tsp pure maple syrup

1 tsp pure vanilla extract

1 tsp baking powder

½ tsp cinnamon

¼ tsp sea salt

Extra Boosts:

Unsweetened shredded coconut, toasted

Handful of fresh berries

Virgin coconut oil, melted

Butter

Pure maple syrup, lightly drizzled

Silver Dollar Vanilla Pancakes

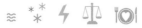

There's nothing quite like dropping a dollop of batter onto a hot, oiled skillet and watching it spread, bubble, and form into a fluffy, golden pancake. Our protein-packed pancakes are so light, naturally sweet, healthy, and super quick to whip up, it makes us wonder why anyone would use a boxed mix these days. We recommend making a double batch of these pancakes so that you have extra on hand in the fridge or freezer. Just reheat in the toaster oven for quick breakfasts, or even for quick snacks on days when you don't feel like being in the kitchen.

1. Place all the ingredients in a food processor or blender and blitz until a liquid, creamy batter forms. Or you can do this by hand by whisking all the ingredients together in a bowl. You may need to use a silicone spatula to remove the batter from your blender or food processor.

2. Heat a skillet over medium heat. Add 2–3 teaspoons of coconut oil and swirl it around.

3. Once heated, drop a little less than ¼ cup of the batter onto the skillet and cook for a few minutes on one side, until the pancake looks as if it's really starting to solidify. Gently wiggle a spatula under the pancake and flip it over. Cook it for a few minutes on the second side, without flattening it. These pancakes tend to burn quickly, so be careful to keep the skillet at a medium heat, and add more oil if the pancakes are beginning to stick. Repeat until all the batter is cooked.

4. Serve topped with toasted coconut, berries, melted coconut oil, butter, or maple syrup, if desired.

continued

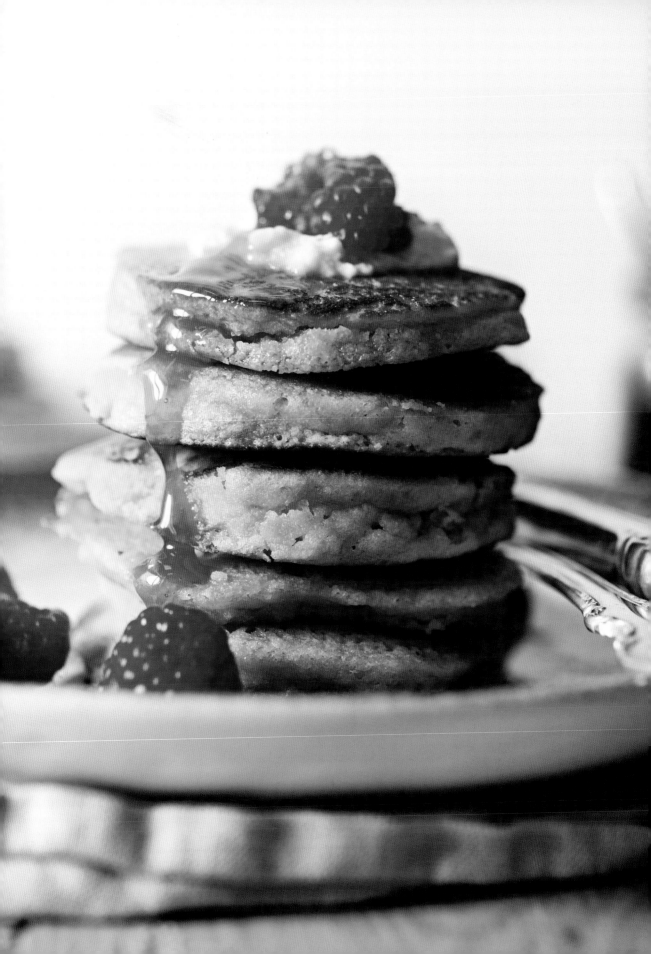

5. Freeze for 2–3 months in an airtight ziplock bag or container, placing a piece of parchment or waxed paper between the pancakes before freezing so that you can easily remove them when you're ready to reheat in the toaster oven. Or keep them in an airtight container in the fridge for up to 1 week.

If you don't feel like standing over a skillet while each pancake cooks, you can use the oven cooking method instead. Preheat your oven to 350°F, spoon the batter into round discs on a baking sheet lined with parchment paper, and bake for 12 to 14 minutes. They'll get an awesome, craggy top but won't get exactly the same golden color as stove-top pancakes.

MAKES 9 MUFFINS

FREEZE: 2–3 MONTHS

PREP TIME: 12 MINUTES

COOK TIME: 25 MINUTES

---

2 ripe bananas, peeled and
    mashed

3 eggs

1 tsp pure vanilla extract

2 Tbsp virgin coconut oil

2 cups blanched almond flour

½ tsp baking powder

½ tsp cinnamon

1 cup fresh blueberries

NUTRITION NOTE Blueberries
are rich in the phytonutrient
resveratrol, which can help slow
the growth of cancer cells.

Blueberry Burst Muffins

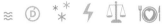

Blueberry muffins were a staple in my household when I was growing up. One day, when I was a kid, my mom found a blueberry muffin recipe in a cookbook and made them. My father criticized the muffins for being too dry, too sweet, and just not up to his standards, to which my mother replied, "Then you make them!" My dad took the challenge seriously, and every week we had fresh, healthy-ish blueberry muffins for breakfast. Now, this recipe is not the one my parents came up with . . . I would argue that it's way, way better. Our muffins burst with tart blueberries and have natural sweetness from almond flour and banana (no refined sugar here!). They're a delightful alternative to traditional, high-carb, sugary muffins, and because they have protein they'll fuel you all morning long. Use these muffins as a snack on treatment days. Thanks to the protein in the almond flour and the healthy fat in the coconut oil, they're filling *and* energizing. **TG**

1. Preheat the oven to 350°F.
2. In a large bowl, mix together the bananas, eggs, and vanilla extract.
3. Melt the coconut oil by placing it in a small pot on the stove top over medium-low heat until it liquefies. Pour it into the banana batter and mix.
4. Add the almond flour, baking powder, and cinnamon, and stir to combine. Then fold in the blueberries.
5. Spoon about ⅓ cup of the batter into each cup of a muffin tin lined with muffin liners and bake for 25 minutes, or until an inserted toothpick comes out clean.
6. These muffins can be stored in an airtight container in the fridge for up to a week and in the freezer for 2–3 months.

Hazelnut flour is a great alternative to almond flour, if you want to switch things up a little.

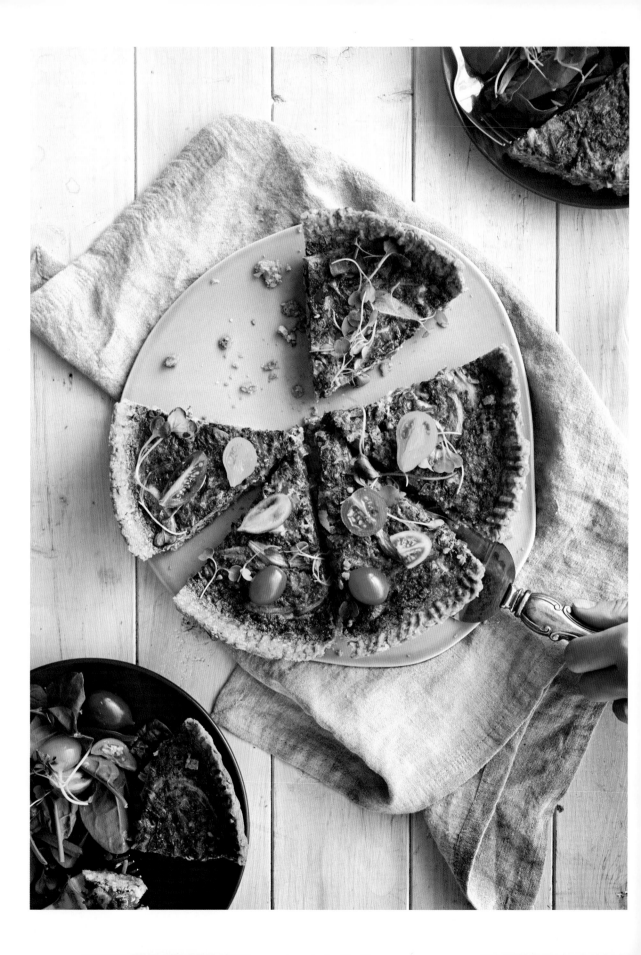

Crust:

1 cup chickpea flour

½ cup rolled oats

3 Tbsp sesame seeds

¼ tsp sea salt

¼ cup water

¼ cup extra-virgin olive oil

Pesto:

1 cup packed basil leaves

¼ cup extra-virgin olive oil

¼ cup raw pine nuts or raw sunflower seeds

2 tsp fresh lemon juice

1 garlic clove

¼ tsp sea salt

Filling:

4 eggs

½ cup unsweetened dairy-free milk

½ cup diced shallots or yellow onion

1 Tbsp extra-virgin olive oil

1 cup chopped spinach

½ cup red pepper, diced

¼ tsp sea salt

Extra Boosts:

⅓ cup halved cherry tomatoes

Small handful of sprouts

Pesto Vegetable Quiche

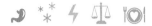

In our opinion, the best part of any quiche or pie is the crust . . . and this crust has it all—it's flaky, crumbly, golden, and nutty. We've made this quiche for clients who are undergoing treatment and needed an alternative to white flour crusts, and everyone always loves it—you will too. You can make this quiche in advance and store it in the fridge to eat for several days. Just reheat it in the oven or toaster oven, and serve it with a small salad or soup, or have it on its own on those days when you can't eat heavier meals. It's perfect for breakfast, lunch, or dinner.

1. Preheat the oven to 350°F.
2. For the crust, in a large bowl mix the chickpea flour, rolled oats, sesame seeds, and salt together. Make a well in the middle of the bowl and pour in the water and olive oil. Use your hands to form the dough into a ball. If it's too dry and won't make a ball, gradually add a few spoonfuls of water until the dough sticks together.
3. Oil a 9-inch pie dish. Place the ball of dough in the middle, and, with your hands, spread it out on the bottom and sides of the dish. Prick a few holes in the dough with a fork to allow steam to escape when baking. Bake for 10 minutes and then remove from the oven.
4. While the crust is baking, make the pesto. Rinse the basil leaves and dry them well, then put all the pesto ingredients in the food processor and pulse until smooth.
5. For the filling, in a medium-sized bowl, whisk together the eggs and milk and set aside.
6. Over medium heat, sauté the shallots in the olive oil for 5 minutes, or until translucent. Then add the spinach, peppers, and sea salt for 1 minute.

continued

7. Let the vegetables cool down slightly, then fold them into the egg mixture with ¼ cup of the pesto.
8. Pour the egg mixture into the pie dish. Bake for 35–45 minutes or until the quiche is firm and the middle is spongy to the touch.
9. Store in an airtight container in the fridge for up to 5 days or in the freezer for 2–3 months.
10. When you're ready to eat, garnish with cherry tomatoes and sprouts if you like.

Simplify this recipe by using store-bought pesto and skipping the step of sautéeing the veggies. Just add them into the egg mixture raw.

If you aren't eating chickpeas or other legumes, you can make this into a frittata instead—omit the crust and cook up the filling.

The pesto recipe makes more than what is needed for the filling, so just freeze the leftover pesto and use it later, or store it in the fridge for up to 4 days, to spread on cooked veggies or noodles.

———————

½ cup steel-cut oats

1½ cups water

½ cup unsweetened dairy-free milk

½ tsp pure vanilla extract

½ tsp cinnamon

¼ tsp ground ginger

Extra Boosts:

Handful of walnuts, pecans, or almonds

Handful of fresh berries

2 Tbsp hemp seeds

2 Tbsp unsweetened shredded coconut

1 tsp slippery elm

Drizzle of pure maple syrup

NUTRITION NOTE Steel-cut oats are made from whole oat groats that have been chopped up into pieces. They are less processed than rolled or quick oats.

Overnight Oats

This is one of our favorite go-to recipes. Not only are overnight oats much richer and creamier than the quick packaged oatmeal that you make in the morning in five minutes or less, but soaking the oats in water overnight increases their digestibility and makes it easier for your body to absorb their nutrients, especially if your digestion is compromised from treatment or cancer itself. Their soft, gentle texture makes this an ideal breakfast for anyone experiencing dry or sore mouth. This oatmeal tastes sweet served with cinnamon and fresh berries, plus it saves time in the morning because it cooks itself overnight.

1. Before you go to bed at night, combine the oats and water in a pot and bring to a boil.
2. Boil for 1 minute and then turn the burner off and cover the pot with a lid.
3. Leave the covered pot sitting on the stove top overnight.
4. When you are ready to eat breakfast in the morning, heat up the oats on the stove and add dairy-free milk, vanilla extract, cinnamon, and ginger to the pot.
5. Top with some of our suggestions, or add your own, and enjoy!

You can make a double batch of this and store in the fridge for up to 5 days to reheat for more breakfasts.

1½ cups unsweetened dairy-free milk

¼ cup chia seeds

1 tsp pure maple syrup

½ tsp pure vanilla extract

¼ tsp cinnamon

⅛ tsp ground ginger

Toppings:

½ cup fresh berries (blackberries, blueberries, roughly chopped strawberries, or raspberries)

3 Tbsp raw Brazil nuts, chopped

2 Tbsp unsweetened shredded coconut

Extra Boosts:

Dairy-free coconut yogurt

Granola

NUTRITION NOTE Chia seeds provide a great source of soluble fiber and can help ease constipation. They are rich in omega-3s, which can help reduce inflammation in your cells.

Chia Coconut Breakfast Pudding

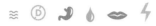

I have to admit that I was wary of chia pudding for a long time, because, like many of our clients, I wasn't sure how to make chia seeds taste good. Well, adding some spices and maple syrup does the trick! I now love opening the fridge door and seeing glass jars filled with chia pudding—it always looks elaborate and fancy, despite how easy it is to prepare. Chia seeds are soft and create a pudding-like texture, which makes this dish easy to eat, especially when you have a sore mouth. And you'll love the way it tastes—with its subtle hints of vanilla and cinnamon, this is the recipe to make when you want a light but delicious breakfast (or snack, or even dessert!). **SG**

1. Whisk together the dairy-free milk with the chia seeds, maple syrup, vanilla extract, cinnamon, and ginger. You'll want to use a whisk, because chia seeds tend to lump together if you use a spoon to stir them.
2. Pour the mixture into a glass container, or portion out into smaller jars, and put on the lids.
3. Let the pudding sit in the fridge for at least 30 minutes or overnight. The mixture will continue to thicken as long as it sits.
4. Top with fresh berries, chopped Brazil nuts, and shredded coconut.
5. If you want to make a parfait, scoop a few tablespoons of chia pudding into a cup or jar. Add a layer of berries and nuts, then top with more of the pudding mixture. Continue to layer until you've almost filled the cup. Top with nuts, coconut, and berries. Add dairy-free coconut yogurt or granola to your last layer, if you want.

You can prepare a double batch of the recipe, portion it out into individual small (8 oz) mason jars, and store it in the fridge for up to 4 days for a delicious and quick breakfast.

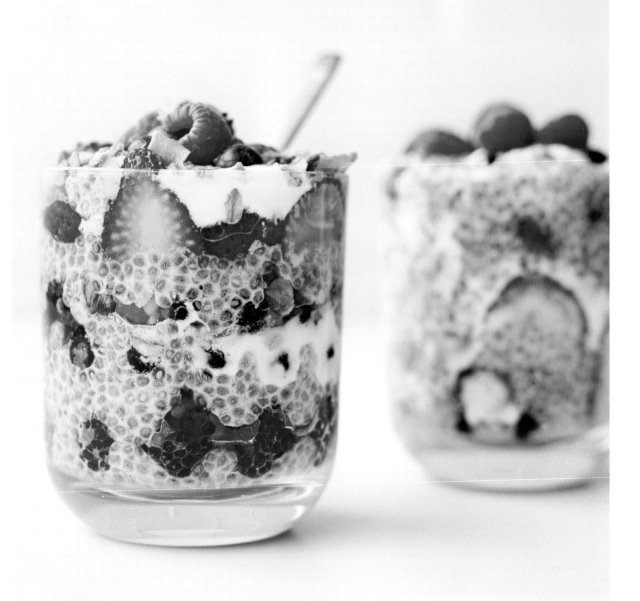

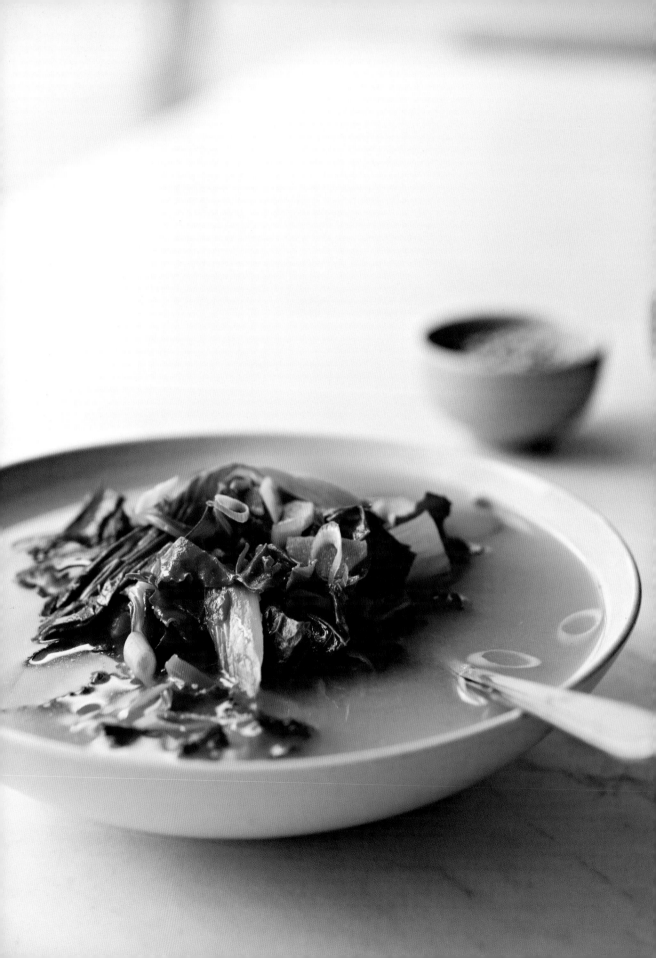

SOUPS

Soups are soothing, warming, and healing; they will become an absolute must as you undergo treatment. They will help you with many side effects, like nausea, dry mouth, low saliva production, trouble swallowing, or loss of appetite. As veggies simmer in broth, they release many of their vitamins and minerals, making soup an easy way to get important nutrients into your diet. The recipes in this section combine a variety of spices, vegetables, and unique flavors to stimulate appetite, relieve nausea, and energize the body. Our three broth recipes are the base for many of our other soups, so we recommend making those first and making a big ol' batch of 'em. But, if you don't have those on hand, a store-bought organic stock or broth will do.

Our Tips for Freezing and Defrosting Soups

Soups are one of the best things to make in advance and freeze so you'll have them ready when you need them. It is best to use frozen soup within three to four months after freezing (broth can be frozen for longer: six to twelve months). To make sure your soups freeze well, follow these tips:

• Leave some space at the top of the container. Liquid expands as it freezes, so leave a little extra room to make sure it doesn't break your container in the freezer.

• Measure out small portions before freezing. It'll be a lot easier to defrost and reheat individual servings of soup. Portion out one or two cups of soup or broth in small containers or sturdy ziplock bags before freezing. Lay the ziplock bags flat in the freezer for easy storing and defrosting.

• Let the soup cool down before freezing, because quick temperature changes are a risk for food safety. You can place the pot of soup in an ice bath to help speed up the cooling process (put ice in a large container or in the sink and then place the pot of soup in that).

• Defrost soup by placing it on a plate in the fridge a day before you want to eat it (the plate will catch any drips). You can also place the frozen bag or container in a bath of warm water.

• Transfer the defrosted (or semi-defrosted) soup to a pot on the stove on medium heat and use a wooden spoon to break up large blocks of frozen soup.

Broths

The three broths we've included here act as the base in all of our soup recipes, but they can also be enjoyed on their own. They're one of the easiest ways to nourish yourself when you have no appetite, feel nauseated, are experiencing dry mouth or low saliva production.

There's no specific way to chop vegetables for these recipes. You can chop them coarsely in large pieces about one to two inches in size. You can leave the skins on all the organic root veggies for added nutrients unless you're using nonorganic vegetables; then it's best to peel them. And, if you can, use organic chicken and bones, because many of the toxins that accumulate in the meat will end up in the broth.

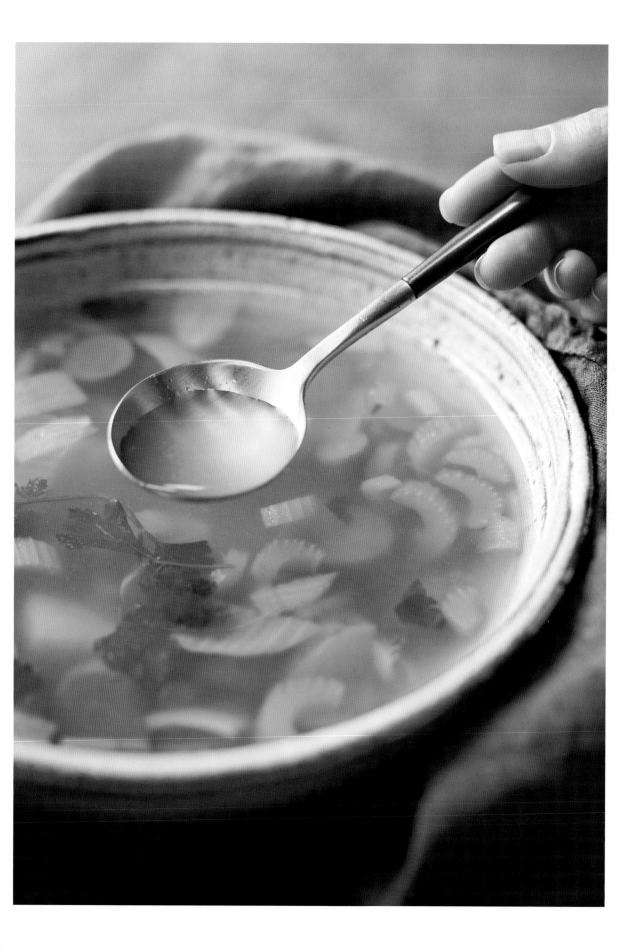

----

1 whole organic chicken
(2–3 pounds)

4 carrots, peeled and chopped

4 celery stalks, chopped

3 parsnips, peeled and chopped

2 yellow onions, chopped

½ bunch fresh parsley

½ bunch fresh dill (optional)

2 bay leaves

2 tsp sea salt

10½ cups water

Organic Chicken Broth

When a recipe gets passed down for generations, you know it has to be really, really good, and this recipe is no exception. My great-grandmother, Bubby Becky, was the originator, and because this recipe needs to be shared, I am now passing it on to you. My hope is that this page in your book will become spattered with splashes of ingredients as you make it. This is the true test of a beloved recipe that is made over and over again. People often refer to chicken broth or soup as "Jewish penicillin" because it's believed to have miraculous healing properties, and it sort of does, with the incredible amount of protein, fat, and minerals all working together to strengthen and heal the body. We use this as the base for many of our other soups, but don't be fooled: it can also be sipped by itself throughout the day or enjoyed by the bowlful. **TG**

1. Place a large stock pot on the stove and add the chicken, vegetables, herbs, and spices.
2. Add the water to the pot and bring to a boil.
3. Cover the pot and reduce heat to a simmer. After half an hour, scoop the foam that collects at the top and discard it. You can use a slotted spoon to do this.
4. After 2½ hours, use a spoon or tongs to pull out the chicken and place it in a bowl.
5. Pour the soup and vegetables through a fine mesh sieve, scraping the vegetables into the sieve to bring out the color.
6. Store in an airtight container in the fridge for up to 4 days or in the freezer for 4–6 months.

If you want a hearty soup, add the vegetables back in at the end of the cooking time. You can also take the meat off the chicken, discard the bones, and throw the meat back into the soup. Or save the meat for other recipes, like Pesto Sweet Potato Chicken Salad on page 136. Feel free to coarsely chop the veggies; nothing needs to be perfect here.

MAKES 12-14 CUPS

FREEZE: 6-12 MONTHS

PREP TIME: 15 MINUTES

COOK TIME: 2 HOURS

---

6 cups chopped yukon gold
    or red potatoes

6 cups chopped carrots

3 cups chopped celery stalks

2 cups chopped yellow onion

1 cup chopped beets (optional)

6 dried shiitake mushrooms

4 cloves garlic, chopped

2 parsnips, chopped

6-inch piece of dried kombu
    seaweed

1 inch ginger root, peeled and
    chopped

1 bunch of parsley

16 cups water

1 tsp sea salt

Phyto Broth

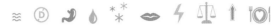

As I was growing up, my dad always made huge batches of vegetable broth whenever anyone in our family was sick. He'd make a day of it—from buying fresh produce to ladling the nutrient-rich stock into glass jars for storage after the delicious-smelling veggies simmered on the stove for the afternoon. To this day I always feel comforted when I smell vegetable broth cooking away in the kitchen, and I hope that you too will find our broth recipe soothing when you have no appetite for anything else. To be honest, you don't have to spend an entire day making this recipe. It's pretty easy to quickly chop veggies, throw them into the pot, and then let them simmer away while you rest. **SG**

1. Put all the vegetables into a large stock pot on the stove and cover with the water. Add the salt.
2. Cover the pot, bring to a boil, and then reduce heat to low and simmer for 2 hours.
3. Allow the broth to cool slightly, then pour it through a colander into another large pot, straining out the vegetables.
4. You can put some of the vegetables back into the broth or eat them separately, if you want. Or enjoy the broth on its own. Add more sea salt to your taste preference.
5. Store in an airtight container in the fridge for up to 5 days or in the freezer for 6–12 months.

Save scraps from other recipes, like broccoli stalks, radish tops and leaves, onion skin, carrot peels, potato skins, and kale stalks, and store them in an airtight bag in the freezer. You can add them to the pot the next time you're making this broth.

If you prefer veggie broth without a pink hue to it, omit the beets from this recipe.

Rinse the vegetables well. It's best to leave the skins on the veggies for this recipe, since they are rich in nutrients. However, if the veggies are not organic, peel them. Chop the veggies coarsely; don't worry about making them a specific shape or size.

---

5 pounds mixed beef bones and meat (marrow, knuckles, neck)

12 cups water

¼ cup apple cider vinegar

3 carrots, peeled and chopped

3 celery stalks, chopped

2 onions, quartered

2 tsp sea salt

2 bay leaves

½ bunch fresh parsley

Strong Bones Broth

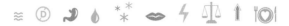

There is a bone broth renaissance that has taken hipsters, health foodies, and everyone in between by storm. Bone broth cafes and bars are popping up around the world and people are ordering cups of broth as they would a cup of coffee. So why the sudden popularity? Well, bone broth is touted as a healing elixir because it contains gelatin and glycine, both of which support the liver, build muscle, supply energy, and rebuild the lining of the digestive tract. Meaning if you have an upset stomach, are feeling nauseated, have a dry mouth, are experiencing weight loss, or have low blood cell counts, it's time to drink Strong Bones Broth. This recipe takes a bit of time to make, but with every brothy spoonful you'll know it was worth it. **TG**

1. Preheat your oven to 350°F.
2. Place all the beef bones and meat on a rimmed baking sheet lined with parchment paper. Make sure the baking sheet is not overcrowded. Roast the meat for 1 hour. You will start to smell the bones roasting before you take them out, and the aroma will be glorious.
3. Once the beef has finished roasting, place a large stockpot on the stove and add all the ingredients.
4. Bring to a boil and skim the foam that slowly floats to the top with a slotted spoon. Reduce the heat, cover, and simmer on low heat for 4–5 hours or up to 12 hours, if you like. You may need to add more water periodically to make sure the bones remain submerged.
5. Allow the broth to cool slightly, then pour it through a fine mesh sieve into another large pot.
6. Store in airtight containers in the fridge for up to 4 days or freeze for 6–12 months in 1-cup portions so it is easy to defrost and use.

MAKES 3 SERVINGS

FREEZE: 3–4 MONTHS

PREP TIME: 7 MINUTES

COOK TIME: 30 MINUTES

---

2 carrots, peeled and diced

1 cup shiitake mushrooms, cleaned, de-stemmed, and chopped

5-inch piece of dried kombu seaweed

1 inch ginger root, peeled and finely chopped

4 cups Phyto Broth (page 119)

2 Tbsp miso

3 Tbsp dried wakame seaweed

1 green onion stalk, finely chopped

½ cup de-stemmed and chopped kale leaves

NUTRITION NOTE This soup is an easy way to eat miso, a fermented soy paste that is especially beneficial for the digestive system and overall immunity. It has also been shown to protect against radiation damage.

Healing Miso Soup

Our version of this soup is immune supportive and more nutritious than what you'll find in a sushi restaurant. You'll taste the savory, sweet, and salty flavors of miso, and the mushrooms, seaweed, and Phyto Broth all add minerals and anti-inflammatory benefits. And if you haven't cooked with seaweed before, this recipe is a great way to try it out.

1. Place the carrots, mushrooms, kombu, and ginger in a medium-sized pot with the Phyto Broth. Cover, bring to a boil, and then reduce to a simmer and cook for 15–20 minutes, until the carrots and mushrooms are soft.
2. Turn off the heat, then ladle ½ cup of the broth into a mug. Mix the miso paste into the mug until it's evenly dissolved, and then pour it back into the pot with the rest of the soup. You can remove the kombu at this point as well.
3. Add the wakame to the soup. Give it a few minutes to expand and rehydrate, and then stir in the green onions and kale.
4. Enjoy right away, or store in the fridge for up to 4 days or in the freezer for 3–4 months.
5. If you're reheating the soup after the miso has been added, be careful to not boil it, as the high heat can destroy the beneficial bacteria found in the miso.

If you don't eat soy, you can buy miso made with chickpeas or other beans at your local health food store or online. We often use white miso because it tastes a bit sweeter than darker varieties, but you can use any type of miso in this recipe.

You'll find the seaweeds at health food stores and online.

Use ¼ cup of dried shiitake mushrooms instead of fresh ones.

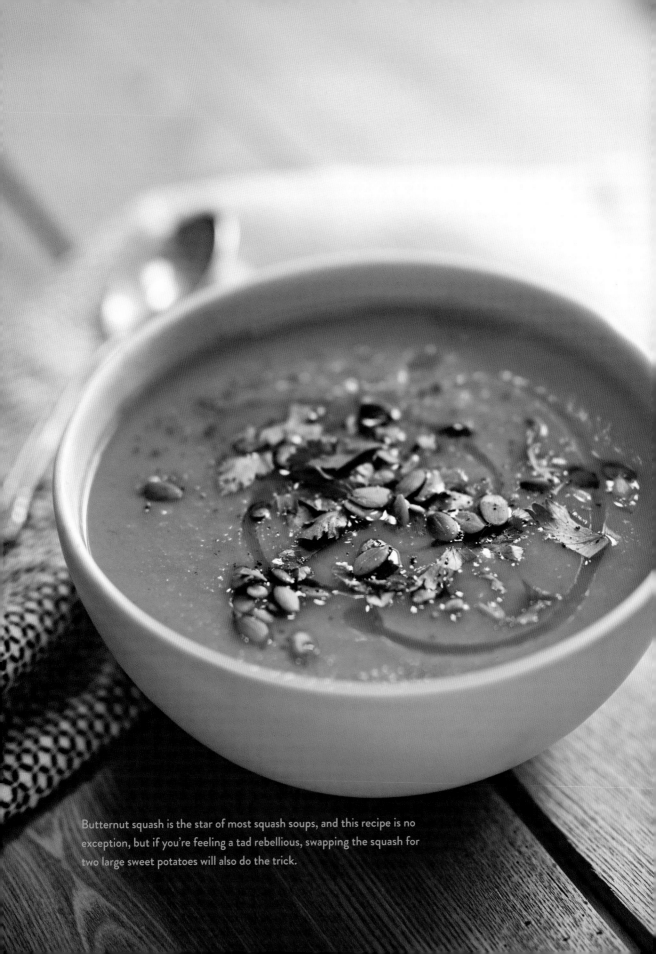

Butternut squash is the star of most squash soups, and this recipe is no exception, but if you're feeling a tad rebellious, swapping the squash for two large sweet potatoes will also do the trick.

MAKES 4–6 SERVINGS

FREEZE: 2–3 MONTHS

PREP TIME: 15 MINUTES

COOK TIME: 40 MINUTES

Soothing Squash Ginger Soup

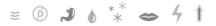

1 Tbsp virgin coconut oil, ghee, or butter

1 yellow onion, cut in half and then quartered

3 cloves garlic, minced

1 Tbsp chopped peeled ginger root

1 tsp turmeric

¾ tsp sea salt

Pinch of pepper

1 butternut squash, peeled, de-seeded, and cut in 2-inch cubes

2 carrots, peeled and chopped in 1-inch rounds

2 Asian pears, peels on, diced

1 sweet potato, peeled and chopped in 2-inch cubes

4½ cups Phyto, Organic Chicken, or Strong Bones Broth (pages 118–120)

Extra Boosts:

3 Tbsp chopped fresh parsley

3 Tbsp pumpkin seeds

2 tsp extra-virgin olive oil

I am a big fan of squash soup, mainly because it was the only soup I knew how to make when I was starting out as a novice cook. It's easy and your final product is consistently good—creamy and golden. I like to find butternut squashes with particularly long necks and shorter bottoms—you get more "meat" from the squash this way without having to scoop out as many seeds. Trust me on this one. This is a great freezer soup and will last in there for 2 to 3 months. **TG**

1. Place a large pot on the stove over medium heat and add the coconut oil.
2. Add the onions and sauté for 5 minutes, or until translucent and soft.
3. Add the garlic and ginger and sauté for 30 seconds, or until fragrant. Add the turmeric, salt, and pepper and coat the onions, garlic, and ginger in the spices, allowing them to lightly cook for about 1 minute.
4. Add the squash, carrots, pears, sweet potato, and broth to the pot and stir well.
5. Cover the pot, bring to a boil, and then reduce to a simmer and cook for 25 minutes, or until all the vegetables are soft.
6. Ladle the soup into a blender or food processor to blend until it's creamy and smooth. (You can also use a hand blender.) Be careful during this step, because the soup will be piping hot. Start blending on low first, hold the blender lid down firmly with a towel and don't overfill it, then incrementally increase the speed.
7. Once blended, season with sea salt and pepper to taste.
8. To serve, top the soup with fresh parsley, pumpkin seeds, and a drizzle of olive oil for added fat and flavor.
9. Enjoy right away or store in the fridge for up to 4 days or in the freezer for 2–3 months.

If you don't have the energy to peel and chop a butternut squash, buy about 4 cups of packaged pre-cubed squash from the grocery store.

---

1 Tbsp virgin coconut oil

1 large yellow onion, diced

3 cloves garlic, minced

1 large bunch of broccoli, chopped into florets and peeled stalks

¼ tsp sea salt

Pinch of pepper

3 cups Phyto, Organic Chicken, or Strong Bones Broth (pages 118–120)

1 cup full-fat coconut milk

3 cups spinach

Extra Boosts:

½ cup cashews, lightly toasted

2 Tbsp unsweetened shredded coconut, lightly toasted

1 green onion, sliced

NUTRITION NOTE The spinach and broccoli offer powerful phytonutrients like beta-carotene, sulforaphane, and indoles, which stimulate DNA repair and break down carcinogens.

Broccoli Coconut Soup

To be honest, I was never excited about cream of broccoli soup: a bowlful of heavy cream and broccoli sounded like a digestive nightmare for my sensitive stomach. Then we swapped in coconut milk, and everything changed for me (and it will for you too). Slowly simmering broccoli, a slightly bitter vegetable, with sweet coconut milk marries two very different flavors to create something exciting, nutritious, and silky. Choose a vibrantly green crown of broccoli and use the whole thing, stalks and all; it adds to the texture and brightens up the green color of the soup. **TG**

1. Place a large pot on the stove and heat the coconut oil over medium heat. Sauté the onions for 5 minutes, until translucent.
2. Toss in the garlic and sauté for another 30 seconds, or until it is fragrant.
3. Add the broccoli florets and peeled stalks to the pot and stir to coat them in the oil, onions, and garlic. Add the salt and pepper.
4. Pour in the broth and coconut milk. Cover the pot, bring to a boil, then reduce to a simmer. Let cook for 20 minutes.
5. Once the broccoli is cooked, add the spinach. It will cook quickly in the hot liquid. Let the soup cool slightly and then carefully pour it into a blender. Blend the soup until creamy. Be careful during this step because the soup will be very hot. Blend on low to start, hold the blender lid down firmly with a towel and don't overfill it, then incrementally increase the speed.
6. Once blended, season with more salt and pepper, to taste.
7. For a bit of texture, fat, and protein, top your soup with lightly toasted cashews, toasted coconut, and green onions before serving.
8. This will keep in the fridge for a few days, and in the freezer for 3–4 months.

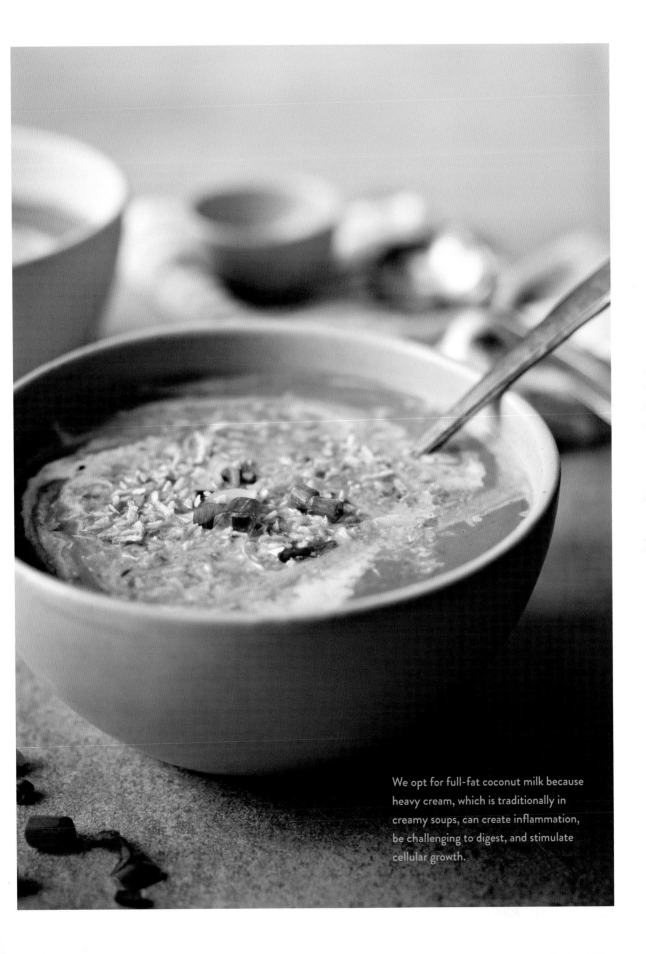

We opt for full-fat coconut milk because
heavy cream, which is traditionally in
creamy soups, can create inflammation,
be challenging to digest, and stimulate
cellular growth.

MAKES 4–6 SERVINGS

FREEZE: 3–4 MONTHS

PREP TIME: 10 MINUTES

COOK TIME: 35 MINUTES

———————

1 Tbsp extra-virgin olive oil

1⅓ cups yellow onion, diced

2 stalks celery, diced

3 cups carrots, peeled and diced

3 cups Phyto, Organic Chicken, or Strong Bones Broth (pages 118–120)

1 cup full-fat coconut milk

28 oz can diced tomatoes

¼ tsp sea salt

Extra Boosts:

¼ cup coarsely chopped fresh basil leaves

2 Tbsp hemp seeds or sunflower seeds

NUTRITION NOTE Lycopene is the phytonutrient that gives tomatoes their bold red color. It protects your cells from damage, but more importantly, research-ers are interested in its possible role in preventing prostate can-cer (and many other types of cancer too).

Creamy Tomato Soup

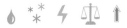

I first made this soup on a whim one winter. My fridge was running low on produce, but there were just enough veggies hiding out in the bottom of the crisper drawer to create a new recipe that has become the go-to, quick, easy-to-make soup whenever my family is short on time but wants something delicious. The simmered tomatoes and carrots naturally taste slightly sweet and, combined with the coconut milk, make a creamy, comforting bowl of goodness that's perfect for cold nights, or when your body could use a little post-treatment care. I highly recommend serving this soup with our Coconut Flour Biscuits (page 215). **SG**

1. Place a large pot on the stove and heat the olive oil over medium. Sauté the onions for 5 minutes, or until translucent.
2. Then add the celery, carrots, broth, coconut milk, diced tomatoes, and salt to the pot. Bring to a boil and reduce to a simmer, cover, and cook on low heat for 25 minutes.
3. Let the soup cool slightly and then carefully pour into a blender. Blend the soup until creamy. Be careful during this step because the soup will be very hot. Start blending on low, hold the blender lid down firmly with a towel and don't overfill it, then incrementally increase the speed.
4. Garnish with basil and serve. Sprinkle hemp seeds or sun-flower seeds on top for extra texture and protein.
5. Store in the fridge for up to 4 days or in the freezer for 2–3 months.

If you don't have coconut milk, you can easily replace it with any other type of dairy-free milk. Just make sure it's unsweetened and plain.

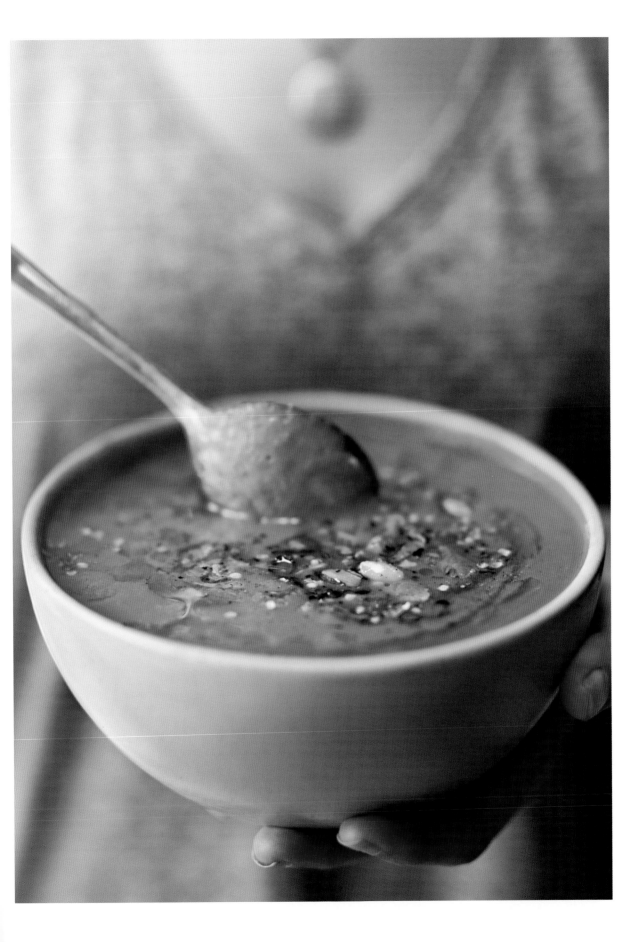

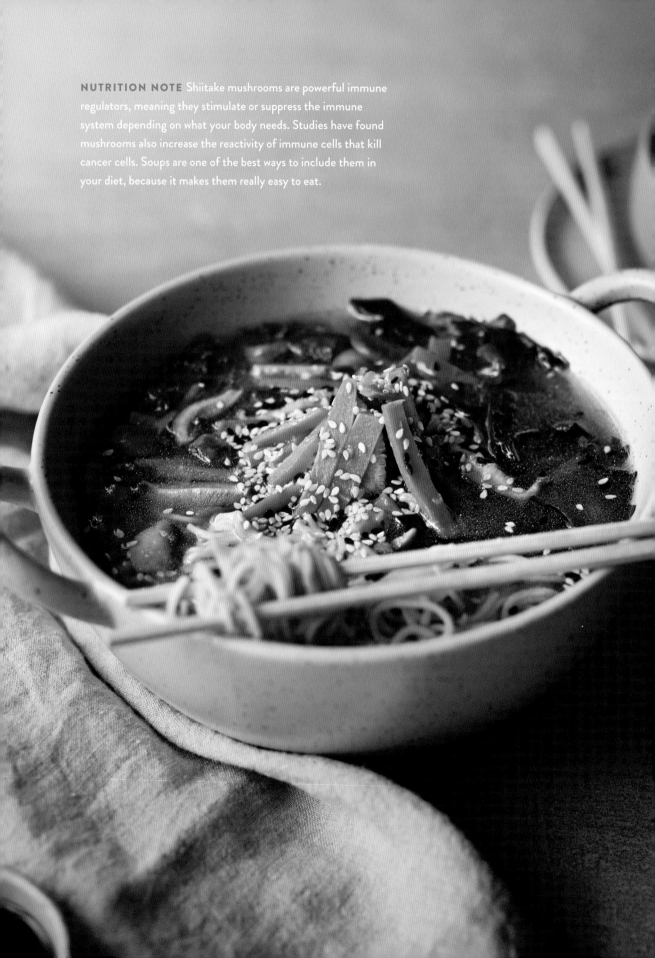

NUTRITION NOTE Shiitake mushrooms are powerful immune regulators, meaning they stimulate or suppress the immune system depending on what your body needs. Studies have found mushrooms also increase the reactivity of immune cells that kill cancer cells. Soups are one of the best ways to include them in your diet, because it makes them really easy to eat.

---

1 Tbsp extra-virgin olive oil

3 green onions, finely chopped
+ 1 tsp for garnish

2 tsp minced peeled ginger root

2 cloves garlic, minced

5-inch piece of dried kombu
seaweed

1 carrot, peeled and sliced

1½ cups shiitake mushrooms,
de-stemmed, cleaned,
and sliced

4 cups Phyto, Organic
Chicken, or Strong Bones
Broth (pages 118–120)

1 Tbsp tamari or coconut
aminos

½ package of gluten-free soba
noodles

2 cups de-stemmed chopped
kale

2 tsp toasted sesame oil

1 tsp sesame seeds

Extra Boost:

1 hard- or soft-boiled egg,
sliced in half

Healthy Ramen

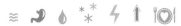

You may think of the sodium-rich, artificial-flavor-laced instant packets of noodles when you hear "ramen." But traditional ramen is an entirely different thing. Our recipe has fresh vegetables and nourishing whole-grain, gluten-free noodles, coming closer to the traditional ramen. There's also mouthwatering spicy ginger and garlic flavors, savory mushrooms, and a subtle hint of aromatic toasted sesame oil. Eat it steaming hot.

1. Place a large pot on the stove over medium heat. Add the oil, green onions, ginger, and garlic, and sauté for 3 minutes.
2. Add the kombu, carrots, mushrooms, broth, and tamari to the pot. Stir well, then cover and bring to a boil. Simmer for 20 minutes.
3. Meanwhile, cook the soba noodles according to the directions on the package.
4. Turn the heat off after simmering the soup and add the cooked noodles and chopped kale to the pot along with the toasted sesame oil. Then ladle into bowls. Top with the reserved sliced green onions, sesame seeds, and egg.
5. Store in the fridge for up to 4 days, with the soba noodles in a separate container (to avoid soggy noodles!). The soup will keep in the freezer for 3–4 months.

Traditionally, the eggs in ramen are soft-boiled, but it's better to fully cook the egg if your immune system is low. If you only have cremini mushrooms, you can use them instead of shiitake.

MAKES 4–5 SERVINGS

FREEZE: 3–4 MONTHS

PREP TIME: 10 MINUTES

COOK TIME: 30 MINUTES

---

1 Tbsp virgin coconut oil

1 small yellow onion, chopped

1½ inches ginger root, peeled and finely chopped

2 cloves garlic, minced

1½ cups de-stemmed, cleaned, and chopped brown cremini mushrooms

2 carrots, peeled and chopped

1 red pepper, chopped

14 oz can full-fat coconut milk

3 cups Phyto, Organic Chicken, or Strong Bones Broth (pages 118–120)

1 cup snow peas, sliced in half lengthwise

¼ cup fresh cilantro, finely chopped

1 lime, juiced

2 tsp tamari or coconut aminos

Extra Protein Boosts:

2 small chicken breasts

Two 5 oz pieces of cod

1 cup cubed organic tofu

Small handful of sprouts

Thai Coconut Soup

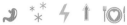

Inspired by our love of Thai food, this soup supplies the body with antioxidant-rich vegetables, and thanks to all the garlic, ginger, and onion, it is full of uplifting flavor and immune-supportive benefits. We like adding lime juice, full of vitamin C, for the immune system, and cilantro, which has antibacterial properties, because they both add an incredible freshness. Enjoy this soup when you have an appetite for something with lots of zest!

1. Place a large pot over medium heat and add the coconut oil and the onions. Sauté the onions for 5 minutes, or until translucent and soft.

2. Add the ginger, garlic, mushrooms, carrots, and red peppers and sauté for 3 minutes.

3. Pour in the coconut milk and broth. If you want to include a protein, add chicken, cod, or tofu.

4. Cover the pot, bring to a boil, and simmer for 25 minutes, or until the vegetables and protein are cooked.

5. Add the snow peas and simmer for 2 more minutes.

6. If you included chicken or cod, remove it from the broth, shred or flake it into small pieces, and put it back into the soup.

7. Top with fresh cilantro, lime juice, and tamari. Add some sprouts, too, if you want.

8. Serve hot. You can store this soup in the refrigerator for 4 days or freeze for 3–4 months.

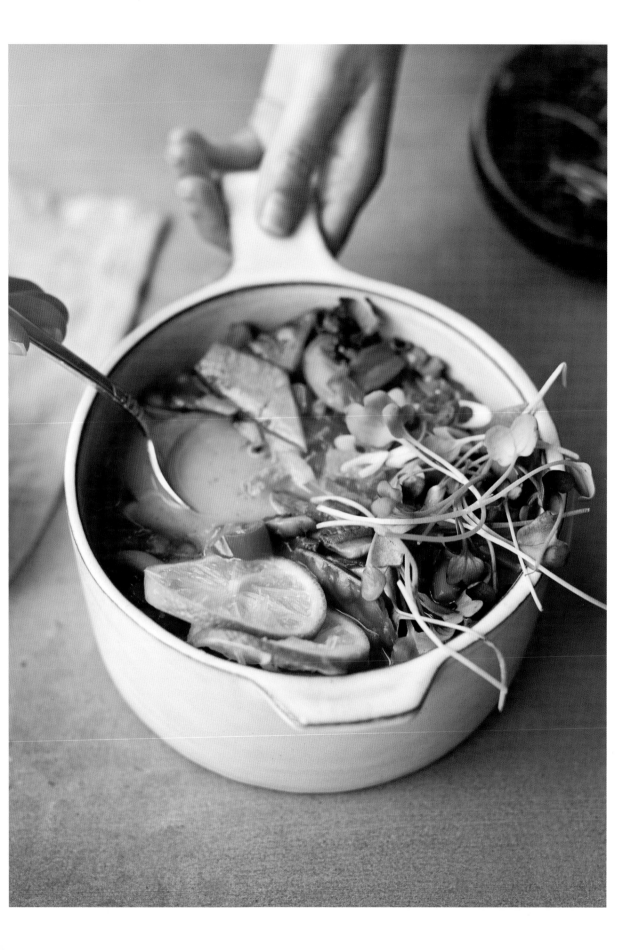

Soup:

1 Tbsp virgin coconut oil

1 cup diced red onion

2 cloves garlic, minced

2 inches ginger root, peeled
and grated

1 tsp coriander

1 tsp turmeric

½ tsp cumin

½ tsp garam masala (optional)

½ tsp sea salt

Pinch of pepper

14.5 oz can diced tomatoes

14 oz can full-fat coconut milk
(set aside 3 Tbsp for the
chutney)

3 cups Phyto, Organic
Chicken, or Strong Bones
Broth (pages 118–120)

3 cups 1-inch cubes of peeled and
de-seeded butternut squash

1 cup dried red lentils, rinsed

Chutney:

½ cup fresh cilantro, loosely
packed

½ cup fresh mint, loosely
packed

⅓ cup unsweetened shredded
coconut, lightly toasted

3 Tbsp full-fat coconut milk

2 tsp honey or maple syrup

1 lime, juiced

Pinch of sea salt

Chutney and Coconut Red Lentil Soup

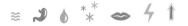

When I was younger, I spent some time in India and did a yoga teacher training course at an ashram there. They made a fresh coconut chutney that tasted out of this world, full of zesty fresh herbs and sweet coconut. Although I've never been able to replicate it exactly, it has inspired this recipe. This soup is comforting when you're feeling tired, and also packed with enough easy-to-digest protein to strengthen your body post-treatment. Our addition of the flavorful chutney takes this soup from basic to bold, but you can always omit this part of the recipe. **SG**

1. For the soup, place a large pot on the stove and heat the coconut oil over medium heat.

2. Add the onions and sauté for 5 minutes, or until translucent and soft.

3. Sauté the garlic, ginger, coriander, turmeric, cumin, garam masala, salt, and pepper. Stir well to coat the onions and garlic in the spices and cook for another minute.

4. Add the diced tomatoes, coconut milk, broth, squash, and lentils, and mix well.

5. Cover the pot, bring to a boil, and then reduce to a simmer. Let cook for 30 minutes, or until the squash and lentils are soft and cooked through.

6. While the soup is simmering, blitz all the chutney ingredients in the food processor until the herbs are finely chopped.

7. Ladle the soup into bowls, scoop about 2 tablespoons of the chutney on top of each bowl of soup, and serve.

8. Store the chutney and soup separately in airtight containers in the fridge for up to 5 days. The soup can also be frozen for 3–4 months. The chutney is best eaten fresh, within 4 days of preparation.

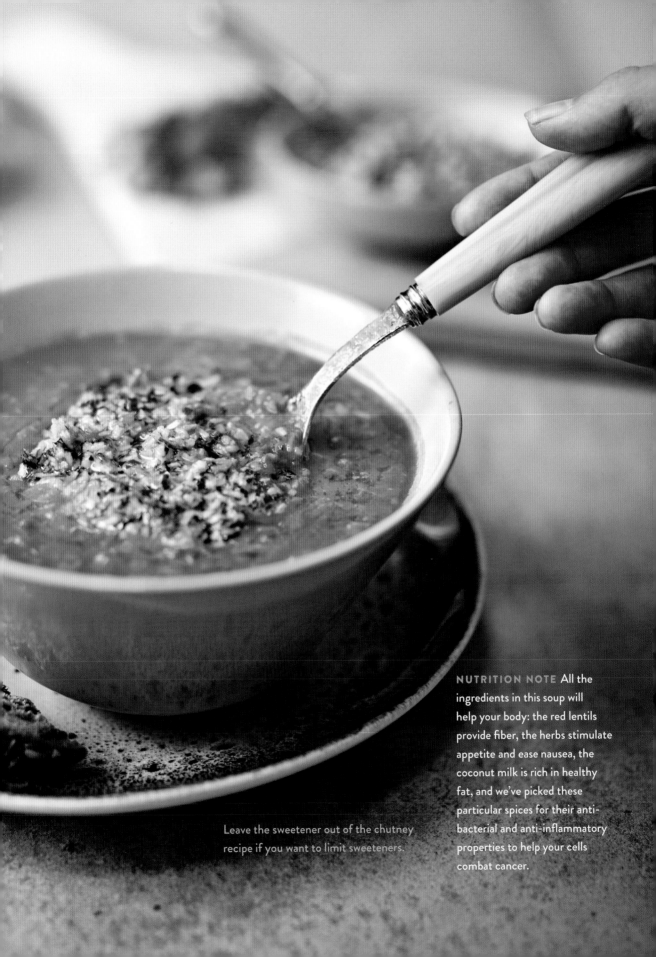

NUTRITION NOTE All the ingredients in this soup will help your body: the red lentils provide fiber, the herbs stimulate appetite and ease nausea, the coconut milk is rich in healthy fat, and we've picked these particular spices for their anti-bacterial and anti-inflammatory properties to help your cells combat cancer.

Leave the sweetener out of the chutney recipe if you want to limit sweeteners.

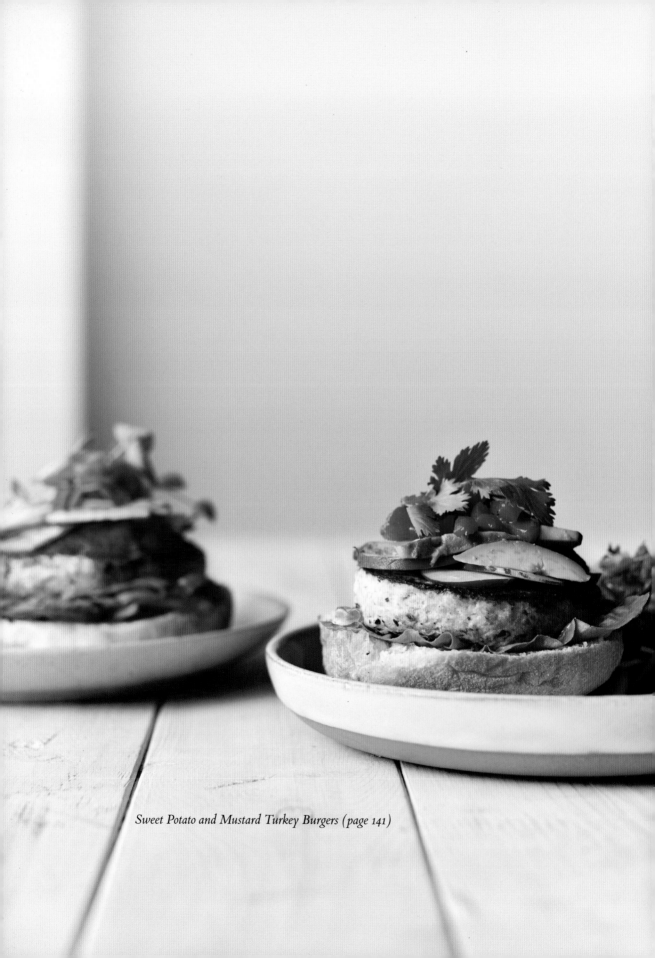

Sweet Potato and Mustard Turkey Burgers (page 141)

OMNIVORE MAINS

This section is composed of all of our animal-protein recipes that include chicken, turkey, and fish. Here, you have a variety of dishes to choose from, from stews to finger foods. Whether you feel like nibbling on something small, like Coconut Chicken Fingers, or eating a big, cozy bowl of Turkey White Bean Stew, we've got you covered.

----

2 sweet potatoes, peeled and
cut into 1-inch cubes

2 Tbsp extra-virgin olive oil

½ tsp granulated garlic powder

¼ tsp sea salt

Pinch of pepper

2 boneless, skinless chicken
breasts

1 cup de-stemmed and finely
chopped kale

1 cup Hempy Pesto (page 243)

Extra Boost:
Handful of sprouts (optional)

Pesto Sweet Potato Chicken Salad

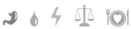

When you combine earthy sweet potatoes with light and lemony pesto, you get an epic potato salad. Then you add chicken, and it gets even better. We know buying pesto is easy, but we highly encourage you to make this one at home. The hemp seeds in the pesto create a creaminess and they provide you with your daily dose of superfoods. Take the time to pull or cut the chicken into small pieces, so that it's easier and gentler to chew and swallow.

1. Preheat the oven to 350°F and line a baking sheet with parchment paper.

2. Put the sweet potato cubes on the baking sheet. Sprinkle with olive oil, garlic powder, salt, and pepper and toss to coat.

3. Roast in the oven for 30 minutes, stirring the sweet potatoes at the 15-minute mark. When cooked, they should be lightly crisp and golden on the outside and soft inside.

4. Meanwhile, put the chicken in a large pot and cover with water and a pinch of salt. Bring to a boil and simmer for 25 minutes. If you have a kitchen thermometer, insert it into the chicken. It should read 165°F or higher. If you don't have a thermometer, cut into the chicken—the meat should appear white with no pink parts.

5. While the sweet potatoes are roasting and the chicken is cooking, make the pesto.

6. Once the chicken is cooked, place it in a colander and run cold water over it to cool it down. Pull the chicken apart with your hands or cut the chicken into small pieces.

7. In a large bowl, toss together the chicken, sweet potatoes, kale, and pesto. Use as a filling for a sandwich or a wrap, have it with a salad or roasted veggies, or simply eat it on its own, garnished with a handful of sprouts.

8. Store in an airtight container in the fridge for up to 4 days.

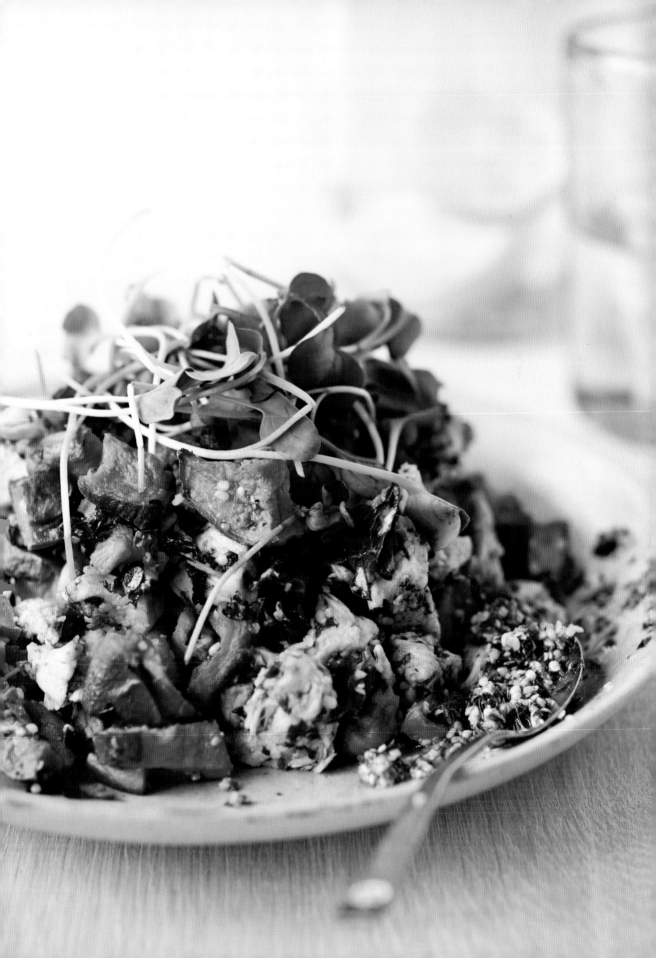

Four 5 oz pieces of cod

2 Tbsp miso

2 Tbsp toasted sesame oil

1½ tsp grated peeled ginger
   root

Extra Boosts:

4 chives, finely chopped

2 tsp sesame seeds

Handful of sprouts (optional)

Miso Sesame Glazed Cod

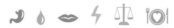

Cooking fish in a miso sesame marinade is super easy and has the most magical results. This recipe is well loved by many of our clients and requires very little effort to make—ideal on treatment days, when you need something quick but tasty. Not only does miso offer a complex flavor that is salty and slightly sweet, and will make your taste buds sing, it also provides naturally occurring healthy bacteria that will support your digestion and immune system. Cooking the fish at a low temperature will help maintain a soft, tender texture that practically melts in your mouth, which is helpful when you're dealing with a sore mouth or throat. **SG**

1. Preheat the oven to 350°F and line a baking sheet with parchment paper. Place the cod on the baking sheet.
2. Mix the miso, sesame oil, and ginger together in a small bowl. Spread some of the mixture over each piece of cod and bake in the oven for 15 minutes. You'll know it's ready when the flesh gently flakes with a fork.
3. Top the cod with chopped chives and sesame seeds and serve. You can keep leftovers in the fridge for up to 4 days and reheat them when you are ready to eat.

There are different types of miso. The darker the color, the saltier and stronger the taste. Lighter misos are less intense, so we recommend you start with these if you haven't used miso before. You can find different varieties at health food stores and online. If you can't eat soy, look for miso that's made with chickpeas or other types of beans.

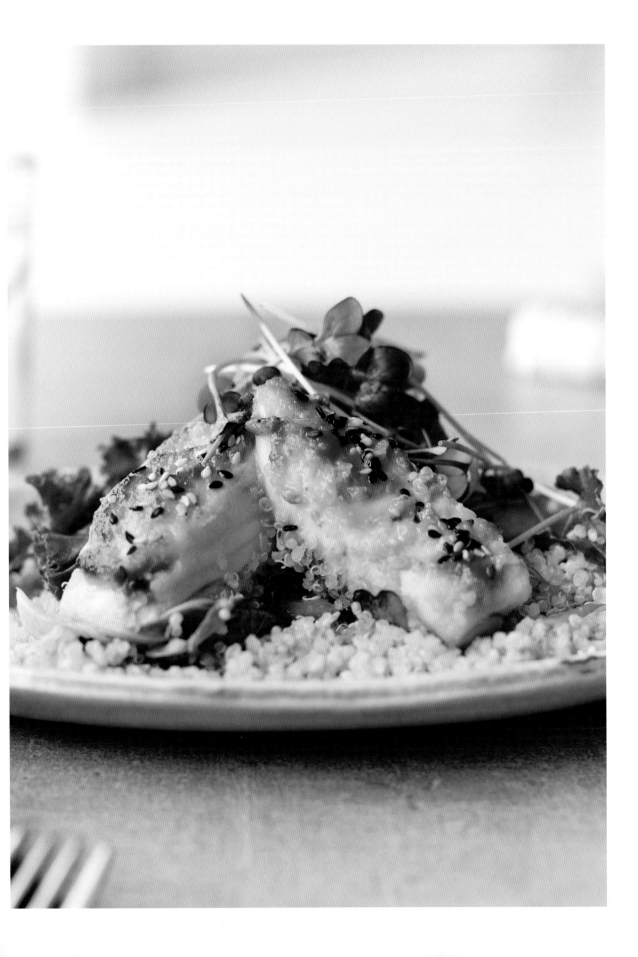

MAKES 6-8 SERVINGS

FREEZE: 2-3 MONTHS

PREP TIME: 10 MINUTES

COOK TIME: 40 MINUTES

Turkey White Bean Stew

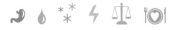

Whenever I am at a loss for what to make for dinner, especially in the colder months, I make this. It's a magical one-pot recipe that's quick, hearty, and satisfying and doesn't require a lot of cleanup—can I get an "Amen"? This recipe makes a lot, so if you freeze it, it can continue to feed you for weeks or months. Top it with freshly diced avocado and *mwah*, perfection! If you're feeling low on energy, with a minimal appetite, a small bowl of this stew is a gentle way to renourish and invigorate. **TG**

---

1 Tbsp extra-virgin olive oil

1 yellow onion, diced

2 cloves garlic, minced

1 lb ground turkey

3 stalks celery, finely diced

2 carrots, peeled and finely diced

2 bay leaves

1 Tbsp dried oregano

2 tsp chili powder

2 tsp cumin

1 tsp paprika

¼ tsp sea salt

Pinch of pepper

4 cups Organic Chicken, Phyto, or Strong Bones Broth (pages 118–120)

14 oz can diced tomatoes

15 oz can white beans, drained, or 1½ cups cooked white beans

1 cup kale, de-stemmed and chopped

½ cup chopped fresh cilantro

Extra Boost:
½–1 avocado, diced

1. Place a large pot over medium heat and pour in the olive oil. Sauté the onions for 5 minutes, or until translucent and soft, then sauté the garlic for 30 seconds.
2. Add the ground turkey, breaking it up with the back of a wooden spoon and brown the meat for about 5 minutes. It's OK if it's not fully cooked through; it will cook further in the stew.
3. Add the celery, carrots, bay leaves, oregano, chili powder, cumin, paprika, salt, and pepper and give it all a good mix.
4. Pour in the broth, diced tomatoes, and white beans. Stir well.
5. Cover the pot, bring the stew to a boil, reduce to a simmer, and cook for 25–30 minutes, or until the turkey is fully cooked.
6. Turn off the heat, and season with sea salt and pepper, if desired.
7. Add the chopped kale, cilantro, and avocado if you're eating it immediately.
8. Omit the avocado and cilantro if it's going in the freezer. Keeps in the freezer for 2–3 months.

½ cup grated yellow onion

1 cup grated peeled sweet
potatoes

1 lb ground turkey

½ cup finely chopped fresh
parsley

⅓ cup spinach, finely chopped

½ cup whole-grain mustard

½ tsp sea salt

Pinch of pepper

NUTRITION NOTE We prefer
to bake our burgers rather than
barbecue or pan-fry them
because baking is the safest
cooking method, creating the
least amount of carcinogens.

Sweet Potato and Mustard Turkey Burgers

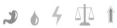

Hands down, these burgers are one of our most popular recipes.
They're moist and juicy and have a savory flavor that comes from
a secret ingredient: a hefty amount of mustard. Half a cup may seem
like a lot of mustard, but believe us, it's what makes these burgers
outstanding. We use sweet potato instead of the more traditional
flour or breadcrumbs, adding extra fiber and supporting DNA repair
to keep your cells healthy during treatment.

1. Preheat the oven to 375°F and line a baking sheet with parchment paper.
2. Use the grating attachment on your food processor and grate
   the onions and sweet potato. You can also do this by hand, with
   a box grater.
3. Mix all the ingredients together in a large bowl until everything
   is well combined.
4. Measure ¼–½ cup of the burger meat and shape into a patty.
   Place on the baking sheet and repeat.
5. Bake in the oven for 25–30 minutes, or until the top begins to
   get slightly golden. You can flip the burgers halfway through the
   cooking time if you want even caramelization on both sides,
   although we always skip this step.
6. These burgers can be stored in an airtight container in the refrigerator for 4 days. You can also make a big batch and keep them
   in the freezer for 3–4 months for a quick meal option.

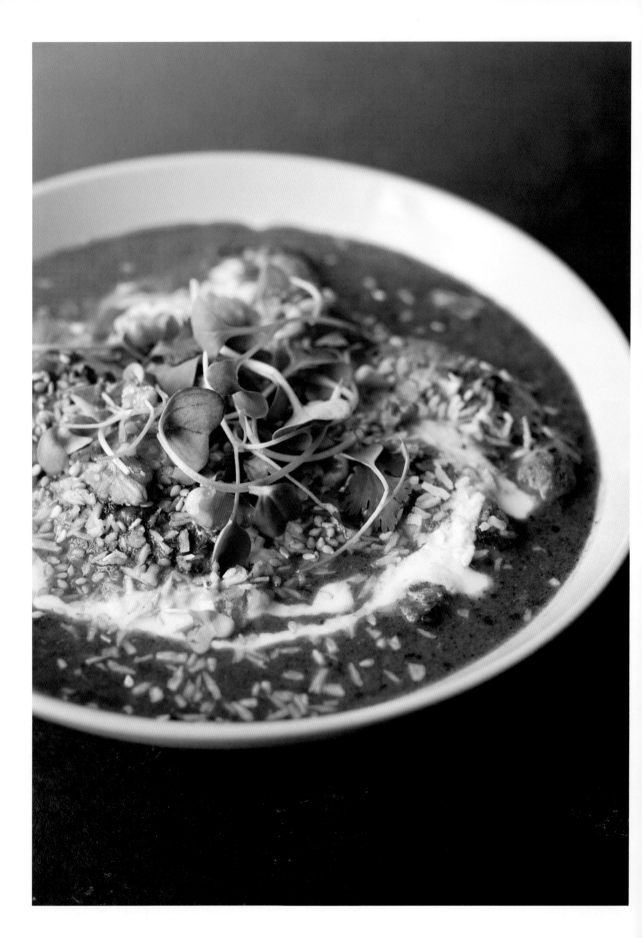

MAKES 2–4 SERVINGS

FREEZE: 2–3 MONTHS

PREP TIME: 10 MINUTES

COOK TIME: 1 HOUR

---

1 Tbsp + 1 tsp virgin coconut oil or ghee, divided

½ cup diced yellow onion

3 cloves garlic, minced

2 tsp minced peeled ginger root

1 tsp turmeric

1 tsp cumin

1 tsp coriander

1 tsp garam masala

½ tsp sea salt

Pinch of pepper

2 cups spinach, coarsely chopped

1 cup kale, de-stemmed and coarsely chopped

⅓ cup fresh cilantro, chopped

14 oz can full-fat coconut milk

4–6 chicken thighs

Optional:
1 cup cooked brown rice

NUTRITION NOTE Leafy greens support the liver in detoxifying carcinogens. They provide fiber as well as minerals, vitamins, and phytonutrients to protect cells. If you're turned off by the color green, you can leave the saag unblended for a golden-colored curry with the same amount of nutritious green goodness.

Saag Coconut Chicken

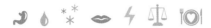

Saag is a traditional Indian curry dish of mustard greens, spinach, and other leafy greens. Although our recipe is a departure from the classic dish you'd find in Indian restaurants, it's still creamy, sweet, and swoon-worthy. Plus, it's gentle on the stomach and all the spices we use have healing properties. The aroma of simmering coconut milk with fragrant spices is enough to make you want to eat the whole pot. If you're not usually a fan of Indian flavors, this dish will change your mind.

1. Heat 1 tablespoon of coconut oil in a wide pan over medium heat. Add the onions and sauté for 5 minutes. Add the garlic, ginger, spices, salt, and pepper and sauté for another minute. Add the spinach, kale, and cilantro, and stir, making sure that all the greens are coated in the spices. Pour in the coconut milk.

2. Simmer for 5 minutes. Take off the heat, then carefully puree in a food processor, until the mixture is perfectly smooth. If you don't have a food processor, use a regular blender, or even a hand blender.

3. Without washing out the pan, add 1 teaspoon of coconut oil to the pan and sear the chicken for 5 minutes per side. Add the blended green mixture back to the pan, cover, and simmer for 30 minutes, or until the chicken is cooked through and has an internal temperature of 165°F or higher.

4. We like to serve this with cooked brown rice, and topped with some sprouts, but it's also filling enough to enjoy on its own, without grains.

5. Store in an airtight container in the fridge, separately from the rice, for 4 days or in the freezer for 2–3 months.

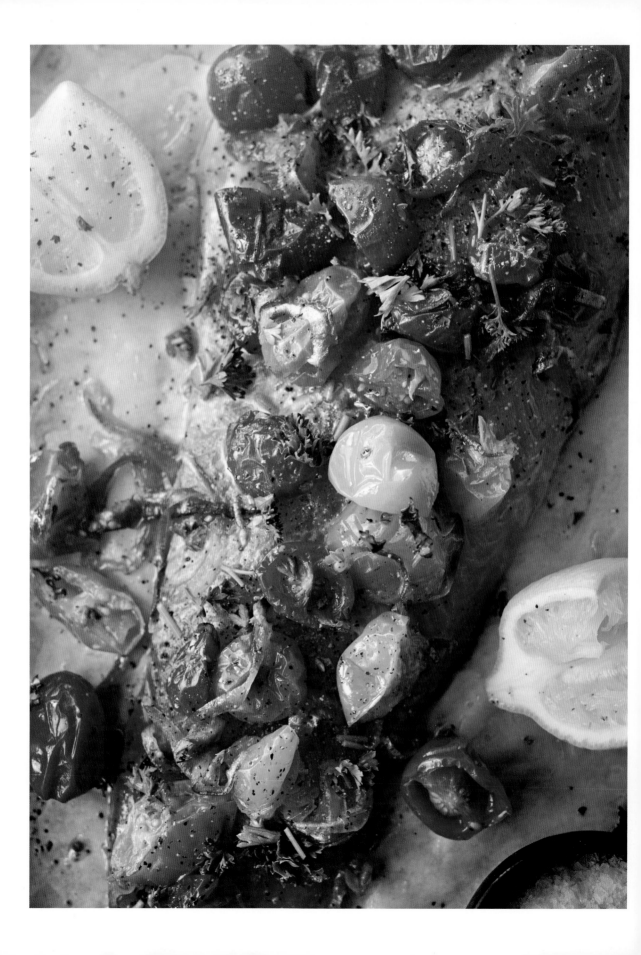

½ cup Rustic Salsa (page 252)

Two 10 oz pieces of trout

¼ tsp sea salt

Pinch of pepper

2 tsp chopped fresh parsley

NUTRITION NOTE Cooked
tomatoes are a wonderful source
of lycopene, a phytonutrient
that prevents free radical damage and has been linked with
reducing and preventing prostate
and many other types of cancer.

NUTRITION NOTE Trout is a
rich source of anti-inflammatory
omega-3s. It also contains
vitamin D, which plays a role
in increasing cancer cell death
and restricting blood supply
to tumors.

Rustic Salsa Trout

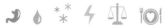

Roasting tomatoes concentrates all the sweetness and delicious flavor inside them, guaranteeing that you'll get the comforting taste of homemade tomato sauce without all the effort, and roasted trout is always a good choice if you dislike "fishy" flavors. When you pair the two, it makes for an uplifting and soothing meal that will leave you feeling full and satisfied, but without any heaviness.

1. Preheat the oven to 350°F.
2. Make the Rustic Salsa.
3. Line a baking dish with parchment paper and place the fish on it, skin side down. Sprinkle salt and pepper over the trout. Then spread the Rustic Salsa over top.
4. Bake in the oven for 15 minutes, or until cooked. Use a fork to gently cut into the center of the fish to make sure it feels tender and flakes apart. You'll know the fish is perfectly cooked when it lightly flakes.
5. Cut the fish into smaller servings. It's best to eat this right away, topped with parsely, but you can keep it in the fridge for up to 3 days and reheat it before eating.

You can prepare the Rustic Salsa in advance.

---

1 Tbsp virgin coconut oil or ghee

1 yellow onion, sliced into thin strips

1 tsp cumin

½ tsp cinnamon

½ tsp turmeric

¼ tsp ground cloves

4 boneless, skinless chicken thighs

Pinch of sea salt and pepper

1 cup dried millet

2½ cups Organic Chicken, Phyto, or Strong Bones Broth (pages 118–120)

1–2 Tbsp fresh lemon juice

1 tsp lemon zest

¼ cup hazelnuts, lightly toasted and coarsely chopped

¼ cup fresh parsley, coarsely chopped

Extra Boost:
⅓ cup pomegranate seeds

Middle Eastern Spiced Chicken

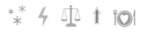

This is a wham-bam one-pot wonder recipe, perfect for when you're going through treatment and have low energy, because there's little cleanup and effort involved. All the ingredients cook together, so every bite is infused with sticky caramelized onions, crunchy hazelnuts, zingy pomegranate, lemony millet, and spiced zested chicken. Toasting the spices in the pan takes away any harshness they have and brightens them right up. You'll be transported to the Middle East without even leaving your kitchen table.

1. Add coconut oil to a large saucepan over medium heat and sauté the onions for 5 minutes, or until translucent and fragrant.
2. Sprinkle the cumin, cinnamon, turmeric, and cloves into the pan and allow them to toast for about 1 minute. Season the chicken thighs with a pinch of salt and pepper and sear the thighs in the pan, about 1 minute per side.
3. Add the millet and broth and stir so everything is dispersed around the pan. Cover the pot and bring to a boil. Then reduce the heat to low and simmer for 30 minutes, or until the chicken and millet are cooked. The chicken should be slightly golden with spices, and it is cooked when the internal temperature reads 165°F or higher.
4. Top with lemon juice, zest, hazelnuts, parsley, and pomegranate seeds.
5. Serve on a big plate or bowl. It's best eaten warm, but you can also store it in an airtight container in the fridge for up to 4 days or in the freezer for 1–2 months.

If you follow a reduced carbohydrate diet, you can easily make this without millet—just omit it and simmer the chicken for 25 minutes. And if you don't have millet on hand but want a carb, swap it for brown rice instead.

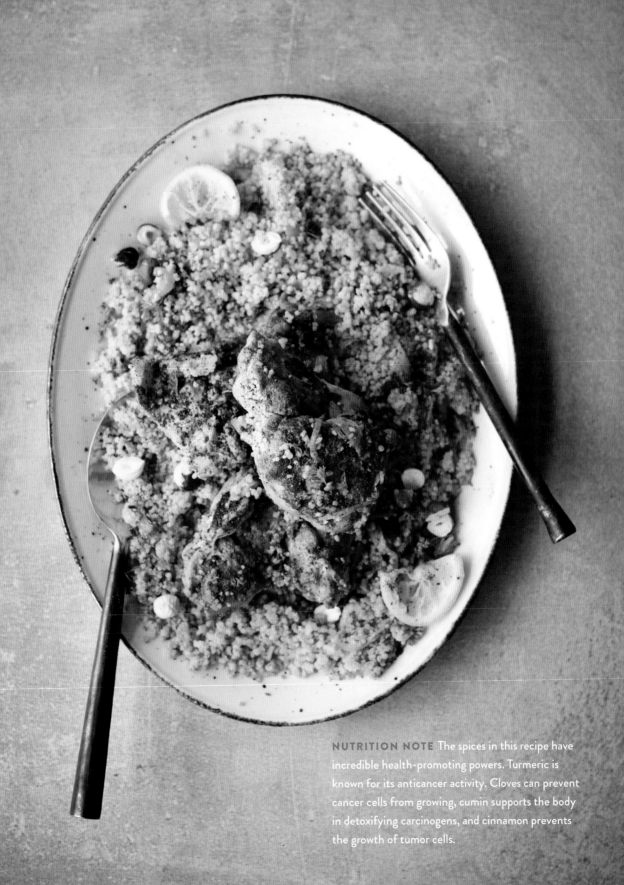

NUTRITION NOTE The spices in this recipe have incredible health-promoting powers. Turmeric is known for its anticancer activity. Cloves can prevent cancer cells from growing, cumin supports the body in detoxifying carcinogens, and cinnamon prevents the growth of tumor cells.

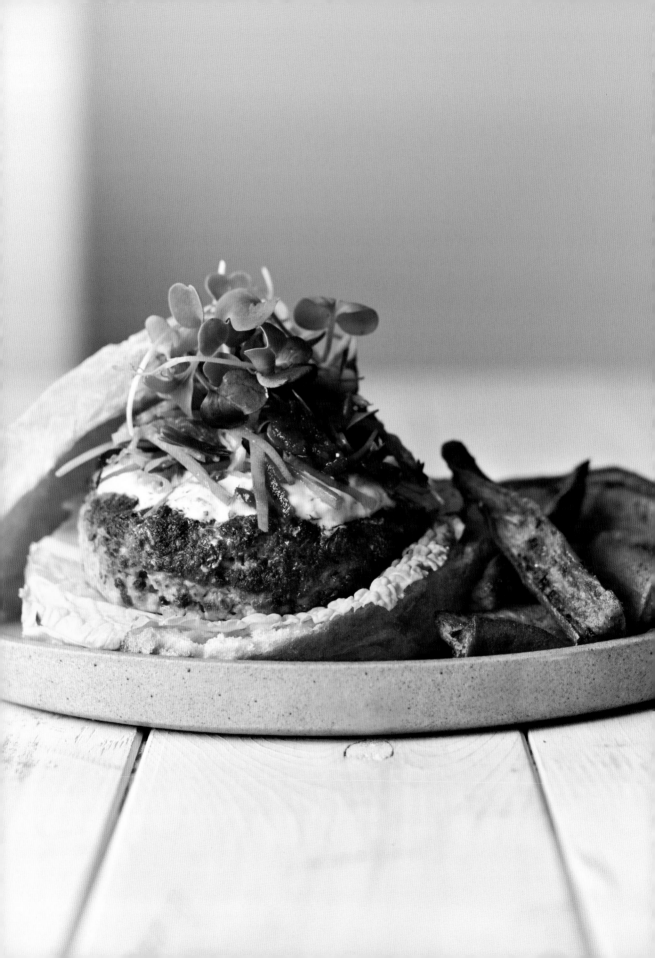

Dill Salmon Burgers

12 oz piece of fresh wild salmon or two 5.6 oz cans boneless wild salmon

½ tsp sea salt

Pinch of pepper

1½ cups cauliflower florets

2 cloves garlic, minced

1 shallot, finely diced

1 egg

½ cup blanched almond flour

3 Tbsp fresh dill, finely chopped

2 Tbsp fresh parsley, finely chopped

1 tsp whole-grain mustard

Coconut Tzatziki (page 244)

Extra Boosts:

Handful of broccoli or sunflower sprouts

Over the Rainbow Slaw (page 188)

NUTRITION NOTE Salmon, especially wild caught, is one of the best types of fish to eat because it contains coenzyme Q10, an antioxidant that reduces inflammation—and reducing inflammation is linked with slowing cancer growth. Salmon also contains vitamin D and selenium, both important nutrients for antioxidant action to protect your cells from cancer.

We made these burgers for all of you out there who don't like the fishy taste of fish. The refreshing dill, vibrant parsley, and sharp garlic and shallots mask the taste of salmon so well that many of our clients eat these burgers every single week. The eggs and mashed cauliflower give the burgers a soft, fluffy texture, which means they're easy to eat. Plus, this recipe is a great way to get more wild-caught salmon into your diet.

1. Preheat the oven to 350°F and line a baking sheet with parchment paper.
2. If you're using fresh wild salmon, place the fillet on a baking sheet skin side down and sprinkle it with the salt and pepper. Bake in the oven for 15 minutes. Once the salmon is baked, set it aside to cool, and then carefully remove the skin. Keep the oven on. If you're using canned salmon, drain the liquid from the cans.
3. While the salmon is baking, put the cauliflower florets in a small pot with ¼ cup of water. Bring to a boil, cover the pot, and simmer for 7–10 minutes, or until the cauliflower is soft and cooked through. Most of the water should be gone by this point; if it is not, drain the excess water using a colander. Then blend the cooked cauliflower in a food processor until it is creamy. If there is just a bit of water left in the pot, you can add it to the food processor with the cauliflower.
4. Crumble the cooked or canned salmon into the food processor, along with the remaining ingredients, except for the Coconut Tzatziki, and pulse to combine. If you don't have a food processor, place all the ingredients together in a bowl and mix by hand.
5. Measure out ¼ cup of the salmon mixture. Shape it into a burger patty, and then place it on the baking sheet. Repeat with the rest of the mixture.

continued

6. Bake the burgers for 20–25 minutes, then carefully flip them over and bake for another 10 minutes. The burgers should be firm to the touch and lightly browned on top when they are ready.

7. While the burgers are in the oven, make the Coconut Tzatziki.

8. Serve burgers with a hearty dollop of tzatziki sauce. Have them in a salad or in a collard or whole-grain wrap, or eat them on their own. You can top them with sprouts and Over the Rainbow sauce if you like. Keep leftover burgers in the fridge for up to 3 days or freeze for 3–4 months.

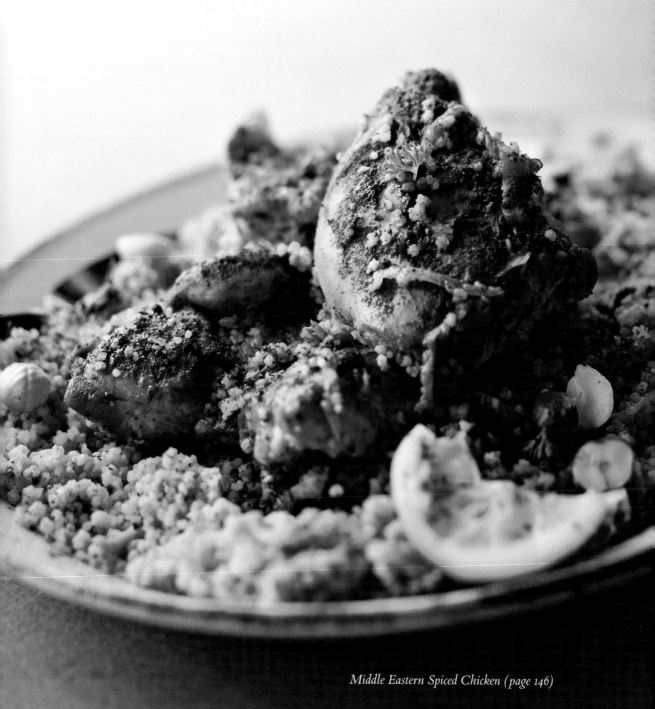

Middle Eastern Spiced Chicken (page 146)

MAKES 2–4 SERVINGS

FREEZE: 2 MONTHS

PREP TIME: 25 MINUTES

COOK TIME: 25 MINUTES

½ cup blanched almond flour
or coconut flour

½ cup unsweetened shredded
coconut

2 tsp Italian seasoning

2 tsp granulated garlic powder

½ tsp sea salt

Pinch of pepper

1 egg

2 boneless, skinless chicken
breasts, sliced into strips

2 tsp extra-virgin olive oil

Coconut Chicken Fingers

As a kid I was a very picky eater, so naturally, I loved chicken fingers (I mean, who doesn't?). But most chicken fingers are deep-fried and pretty unhealthy. So when I needed to get my chicken-finger fix, we came up with this recipe: the best part is they're actually good for you! Instead of panko, we use a combination of almond flour and shredded coconut, which achieves that crispy texture while also adding a bit of natural sweetness and nuttiness. Chicken fingers are fairly manageable to eat when you're going through treatment, and they make a great meal or snack. If you like dips or need some extra sauce, pair them with our Hempy Pesto (page 243) or Coconut Tzatziki (page 244). **TG**

1. Preheat the oven to 375°F and line a baking sheet with parchment paper.
2. In a wide, shallow dish, combine the almond flour, shredded coconut, Italian seasoning, garlic powder, salt, and pepper.
3. In a medium-sized bowl, crack the egg and whisk it.
4. Keep the dish and bowl close together to avoid spillage. Dip each chicken strip into the egg and shake off excess liquid, then dredge it in the coconut mixture and place it on the baking sheet. If some egg finds its way into the dish with the shredded coconut, and the mixture becomes too sticky, simply add about ¼–½ cup more coconut to the mix.
5. Drizzle a little oil over the chicken fingers, then bake in the oven for 25 minutes, or until golden, flipping them halfway through the cooking time.
6. Store in an airtight container in the fridge for up to 4 days or in the freezer for up to 2 months.

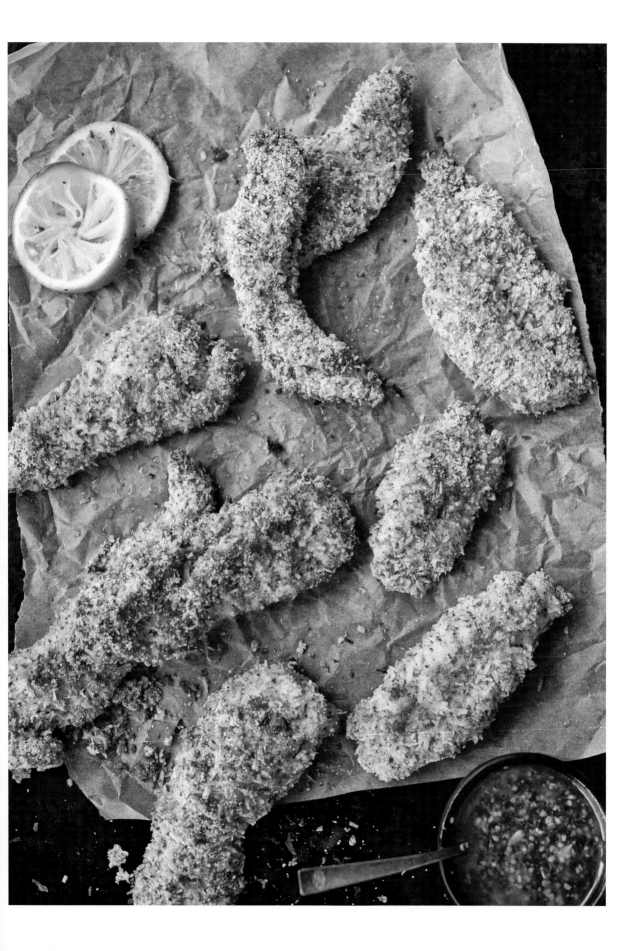

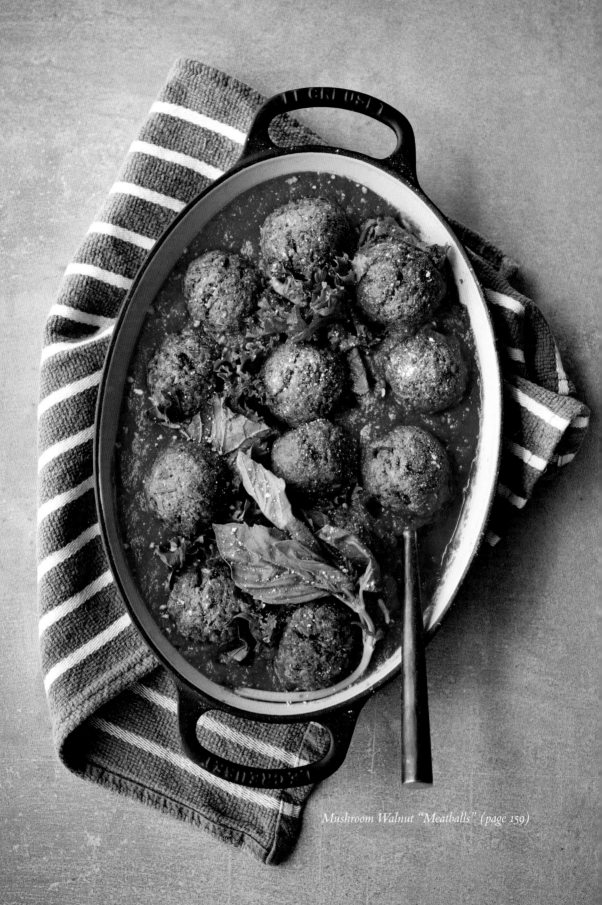

Mushroom Walnut "Meatballs" (page 159)

VEGETARIAN MAINS

Whether you're vegetarian or not, you're going to love these recipes. All of these dishes are designed to include a variety of plant-based ingredients to ensure that you get plenty of easy-to-digest protein and healthy fats. Like our omnivore mains, we've got little bites to nibble on, like our Easy Falafels or more hearty, one-pot dishes like our Lentil Shepherd's Pie and Stewed Coconut, Tomato, and Chickpeas. There are a lot of flavorful options to choose from.

MAKES 8 SMALL OR 4 LARGE
BURGERS

FREEZE: 4–5 MONTHS

PREP TIME: 20 MINUTES

COOK TIME: 50 MINUTES

———————

¼ cup quinoa

1¾ cups chopped peeled sweet
    potato

½ cup diced red onion

2 cloves garlic, chopped

1 tsp paprika

1 tsp granulated garlic powder

½ tsp cumin

½ tsp chili powder

½ tsp sea salt

Pinch of cayenne (optional)

Pinch of pepper

½ cup de-stemmed and
    chopped kale

¼ cup chopped fresh cilantro

15 oz can black beans, drained
    and rinsed, or 1¾ cups
    cooked black beans

1 egg or 1 vegan egg (see recipe
    note)

1 Tbsp extra-virgin olive oil

Extra Boosts:
Avocado

Handful of broccoli or
    sunflower sprouts

Black Bean Tex Mex Burgers

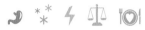

Black beans and sweet potatoes are one of our favorite combinations—just the right amount of both naturally sweet and savory flavors enhanced by mouthwatering spices. Veggie burgers are one of the best items to keep around during treatment; they're easy to make, easy to freeze, and packed with vegetables, and they make a fabulous portable meal or snack. These burgers get their Southwest flavor from a roster of spices, and the black beans, along with sweet potato, kale, and quinoa, make the perfect medley for a hearty burger with a bit of kick.

1. Cook the quinoa with ½ cup of water in a small pot. Bring to a boil, cover, and then reduce to a simmer for 15 minutes. When cooked, the quinoa will be fluffy and the water will be absorbed. Set aside.

2. Preheat the oven to 350°F and line a baking sheet with parchment paper.

3. Use the S blade in a food processor to pulse the sweet potato, onions, garlic, paprika, garlic powder, cumin, chili powder, salt, cayenne, and pepper until a crumbly texture forms. If you're doing this by hand, grate the sweet potato, finely dice the onion, mince the garlic, and place them in a bowl with the spices.

4. Add the kale, cilantro, and beans to the food processor and pulse until everything is combined. Some of the beans should still be slightly intact to add texture, so don't over-process. You can also do this step by hand, using a potato masher or fork.

5. Mix in the quinoa and then fold in the egg.

6. Take ¼ cup of the mixture and form it into a patty. Place the patty on the baking sheet and repeat with the remaining bean mixture. You should have 8 small burgers, but you can also make 4 large ones.

continued

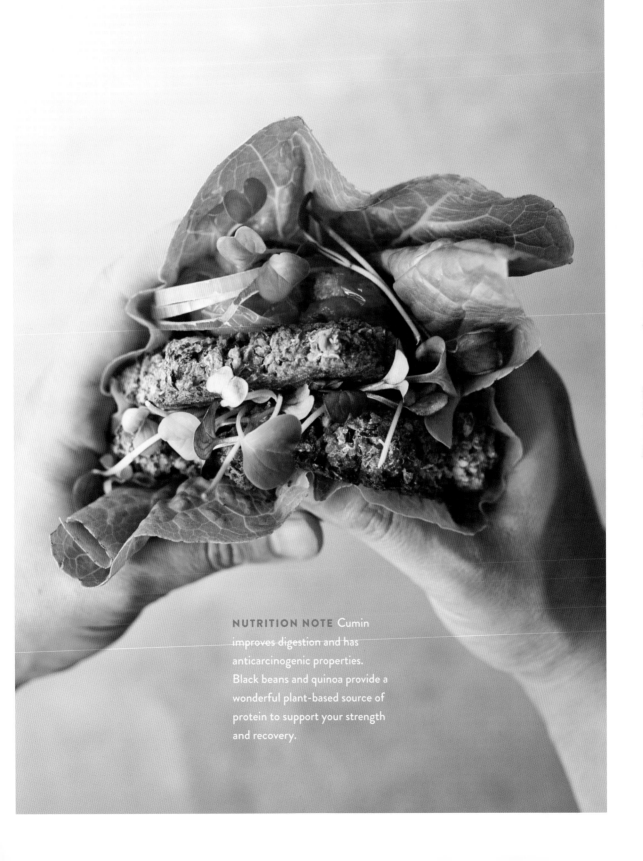

NUTRITION NOTE Cumin improves digestion and has anticarcinogenic properties. Black beans and quinoa provide a wonderful plant-based source of protein to support your strength and recovery.

7. Drizzle the olive oil over the patties and bake for 30–35 minutes, or until slightly crisp on the outside. If you like an even crisp on each side, flip halfway through the cooking time.
8. Eat the burgers as they are or top with some avocado and a handful of broccoli or sunflower sprouts. These can be kept in the fridge for up to 4 days or frozen for 4–5 months.

To make a vegan egg, mix 1 Tbsp of chia or ground flaxseeds with 3 Tbsp of water. Allow to rest for 10 minutes, or until it becomes gelatinous.

MAKES 12 "MEATBALLS"

FREEZE: 4–5 MONTHS

PREP TIME: 20 MINUTES

COOK TIME: 25 MINUTES

---

1 Tbsp chia seeds

1 cup shiitake mushrooms, coarsely chopped

1 cup cremini mushrooms

1 cup toasted walnuts

⅓ cup yellow onion, diced

¼ cup chopped fresh parsley

2 tsp balsamic vinegar

2 tsp Italian seasoning

1 tsp granulated garlic powder

½ tsp sea salt

Pinch of pepper

1 cup brown rice flour

1 Tbsp extra-virgin olive oil

Optional:

Marinara sauce

Gluten-free pasta

Mushroom Walnut "Meatballs"

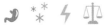

If you don't eat meat, or if you're looking to up your shiitake mushroom game, these "meatballs" are for you—plus, they're great grab-and-go's when you need something that's easy to pack. The mushrooms lend an earthy, almost meaty, flavor, and the walnuts add a nuttiness and slight sweetness. Serve them stewed in homemade marinara sauce (or a good-quality jarred sauce will do the trick) for a completely filling and satisfying meal.

1. Preheat the oven to 375°F and line a baking sheet with parchment paper.
2. Make a "chia egg" by combining the chia seeds with 3 tablespoons of water in a small bowl. Set aside for 10 minutes for the mixture to thicken.
3. Place all the ingredients except the chia egg, flour, and olive oil in the food processor. Pulse until all the ingredients are combined and coarsely chopped.
4. Transfer this mixture to a mixing bowl and fold in the chia egg and flour.
5. Take 2 tablespoons of the mixture, shape into a ball, and place it on the baking sheet. Repeat to make 12 balls.
6. Lightly brush each ball with olive oil.
7. Bake in the oven for 25 minutes.
8. Once they're baked, heat up your favorite marinara sauce and cover the meatballs. You could also make some gluten-free pasta to serve the meatballs over. Or you can simply enjoy them without any sauce. They are also delicious served over a salad or with some cooked veggies on the side.
9. You can store the leftover meatballs in the fridge for up to 5 days. You can also freeze these for 4–5 months and reheat when you are ready to eat them.

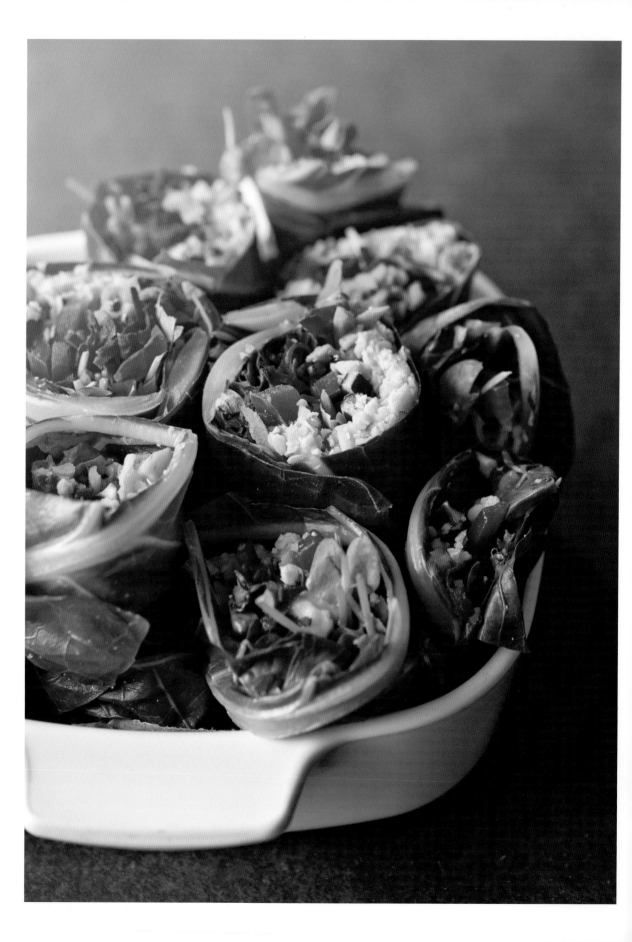

Tahini Tamari Swirl (page 242)

6 collard leaves, de-stemmed

½ cup cooked chickpeas, lightly mashed

½ avocado, sliced

½ red pepper, julienned

½ cup grated peeled beet

½ cup grated peeled carrot

½ cup kale, de-stemmed thinly sliced

½ cup thinly sliced purple cabbage

½ cup broccoli sprouts (optional)

6 fresh mint leaves, chopped

6 fresh basil leaves, chopped

We've chosen to use our delicious Tahini Tamari Swirl marinade (page 242) to give these wraps flavor. But, if you're in the mood for pesto or even hummus, use one of those instead. Flip over to our sauces, marinades, and dressings section (page 241) to pick out one that calls to you.

Rainbow Wraps

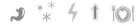

This is the ultimate wrap! Crunchy sweet carrots and beets go perfectly with the crisp of fresh red peppers, refreshing mint, and earthy basil; add some creamy avocado and you've got an explosion of flavor. It's bursting with color, which means the phytonutrient content is high, and the variety of vegetables makes this meal a wonderful energy booster. The thought of using a green leaf as a wrap may be new for you, but it's an excellent way to add cruciferous greens to your diet, especially if you are trying out gluten-free or grain-free options. These are hearty wraps, so make them when your appetite is strong.

1. Prepare the Tahini Tamari Swirl marinade.
2. Slide your knife along the edge of the stems in the middle of the collard leaves and gently cut out the stem.
3. To assemble the wraps, place one leaf down on the counter and place another leaf over it facing the opposite direction, so that the areas where the stems were overlap each other. The tops of the collard leaves should face opposite directions.
4. Spoon 1 heaping tablespoon of Tahini Tamari Swirl on each pair of leaves and spread it evenly to cover the center of the collard leaves. Add 2 tablespoons of the mashed chickpeas in the center of the two leaves, then top with a handful of each of the vegetables in the center. Sprinkle with the herbs. Tightly roll in the top, then the two sides, then the bottom, and slice in half. If your wraps aren't sticking together, you can use a toothpick to keep them closed. These are best served right away, but can also be stored in the fridge for up to 2 days.

If your stomach can't tolerate raw collard leaves, you can lightly steam the de-stemmed leaves (step 2) in ¼ cup of water for a quick 60 seconds. This will make them easier to digest.

MAKES 4 SERVINGS

FREEZE: 2-3 MONTHS

PREP TIME: 10 MINUTES

COOK TIME: 35 MINUTES

----

2 tsp virgin coconut oil

½ cup diced yellow onion

3 cloves garlic, minced

1 tsp minced peeled ginger root

2 tsp turmeric

1 tsp coriander

½ tsp cinnamon

½ tsp sea salt

Pinch of pepper

1 sweet potato, peeled and
diced into 1-inch cubes

2 carrots, peeled and cut into
½-inch-thick circles

15 oz can chickpeas, drained
and rinsed, or 1½ cups
cooked chickpeas

14.5 oz can diced tomatoes

½ cup full-fat coconut milk

2 cups baby spinach

¼ cup chopped fresh cilantro

Optional:
1 cup cooked quinoa, millet,
or rice

Stewed Coconut, Tomato, and Chickpeas

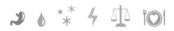

When you need to feel cozy and toasty, make this recipe. A stew is
the perfect dish to cook when you need something filling, quick,
and comforting. This is a great recipe to freeze and reheat after a
day at the hospital, when you need a warming meal to pick you
up. Tomatoes and coconut are a classic duo and when married with
South Asian spices, a really tasty stew comes to life. Chickpeas,
carrots, and sweet potatoes thicken the dish and add to the already
gorgeous orange-reddish color. Garnish with cilantro and spinach
for an extra oomph of freshness.

1. Place a medium-sized pot on the stove over medium heat.
   Add the coconut oil and sauté the onions for 3 minutes. Then
   add the garlic, ginger, turmeric, coriander, cinnamon, salt, and
   pepper and sauté for another minute.

2. Add the sweet potatoes, carrots, and chickpeas and toss around
   so they get coated in the spices.

3. Pour in the diced tomatoes and coconut milk.

4. Bring to a boil, cover, and allow to simmer for 30 minutes.
   You don't need to stir it; just let it do its thing.

5. At the 30-minute mark, drop the spinach into the pot and turn
   off the heat.

6. Serve hot, garnished with fresh cilantro. If you like, serve over
   quinoa, rice, or millet.

7. Place in an airtight container in the fridge for up to 5 days or
   in the freezer for 2–3 months.

We like to pair this with a grain, although it's not necessary. Quinoa, brown
rice, or millet work remarkably well. Cook these grains separately at the same
time as the stew so they can be ready together.

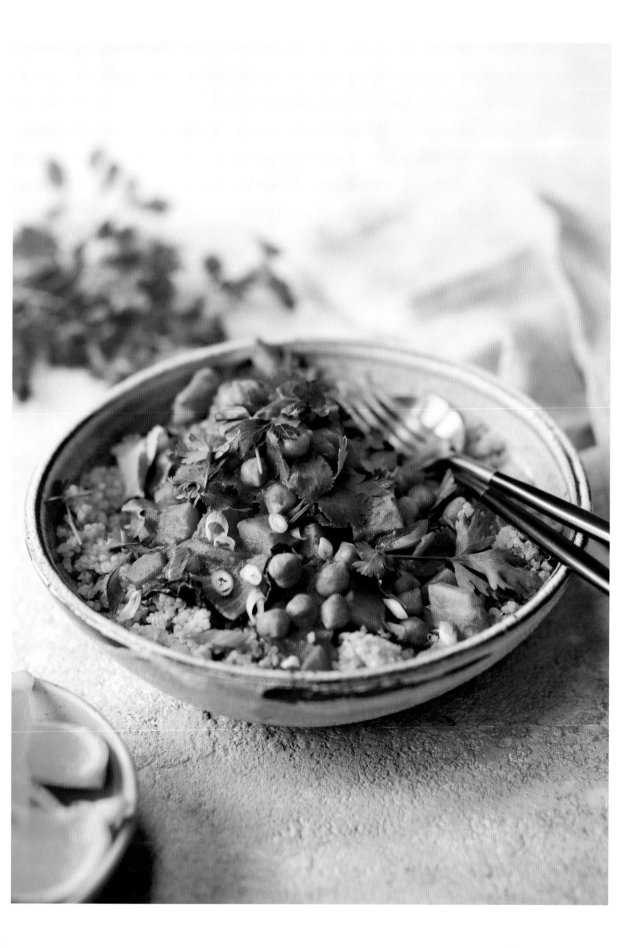

½ cup dried short-grain brown rice, wild rice, or quinoa

2 cups broccoli florets

½ cup Almond Coconut Lime Sauce (page 246)

2 cups cooked adzuki beans

½ cup carrot matchsticks

½ cup cucumber matchsticks

2 radishes, thinly sliced

½ avocado, sliced

1 nori sheet, cut into matchsticks

Extra Boosts:

1 green onion, thinly sliced

¼ cup coarsely chopped fresh cilantro

1 Tbsp sesame seeds

NUTRITION NOTE The adzuki bean is a little red legume that originated in Asia. These are often used in Asian desserts and savory dishes. Like most beans and legumes, they contain a significant amount of fiber, protein, B vitamins, and minerals.

Simple Sushi Bowl

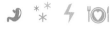

Think of this bowl as a deconstructed roll of sushi, with all of those beautiful, delicious ingredients (that are normally rolled up in nori) shown off. This recipe has everything going for it: creamy avocados, crunchy cucumbers and carrots, and fiber-rich brown rice. There's also another ingredient in here, a powerhouse legume that many people have not heard of: the adzuki bean. When all combined together with our yummy Almond Coconut Lime Sauce, this is a delicious one-bowl meal.

1. Cook the brown rice with 1 cup of water in a small pot. Bring to a boil, cover, and reduce to a simmer for 30 minutes, or until the rice is fluffy and soft and the water has been absorbed.

2. In a small pot, place the broccoli and ¼ cup of water. Bring to a simmer, then cover the pot. Steam the broccoli for 3 minutes. Drain and set aside.

3. Make the Almond Coconut Lime Sauce.

4. Divide the rice between two bowls and add 1 cup of the adzuki beans to each one. Layer the carrot, cucumber, radishes, avocado, and nori on top, along with the extra boosts, if using. Finish it with a drizzle of the sauce.

5. This is best eaten right away, but you can always keep it in the fridge for up to 4 days. If you are storing this in the fridge, add the fresh avocado and nori right before eating.

If you are using wild rice, bring it to a boil, cover, and simmer it for 45 minutes. If you're cooking quinoa, bring it to a boil, cover, and simmer it for 15 minutes.

If you're not strictly vegetarian, you can add a piece of baked or seared salmon to this dish.

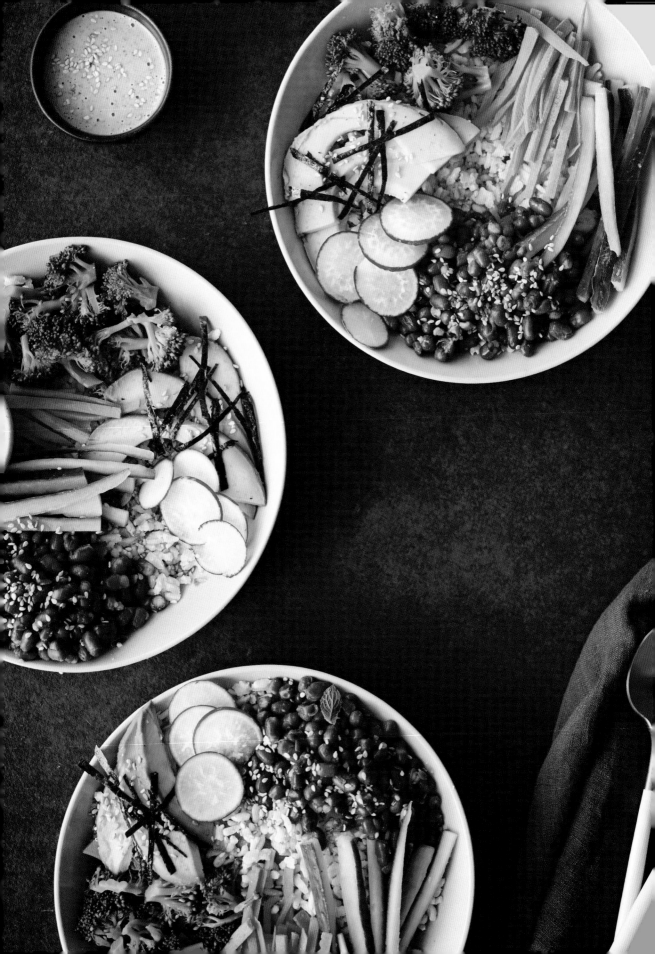

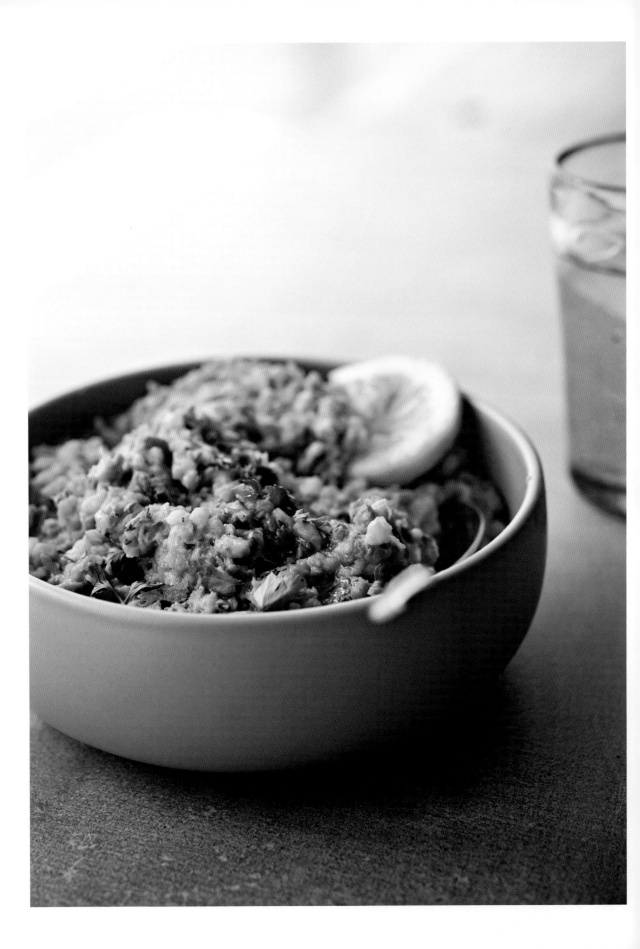

MAKES 6 SERVINGS

FREEZE: 4–5 MONTHS

PREP TIME: 8 HOURS

COOK TIME: 1 HOUR AND

10 MINUTES

---

1 cup dried mung beans

1 Tbsp ghee or virgin coconut oil

2 bay leaves

½ tsp turmeric

½ tsp cumin seeds

½ tsp coriander

½ tsp sea salt

½ cup diced yellow onion

2 tsp minced peeled ginger root

½ cup short-grain brown rice

2 carrots, peeled and chopped into 1-inch pieces

2 celery stalks, chopped into 1-inch slices

½ cup 1-inch cubes of peeled butternut squash or sweet potato

4 cups water or Phyto Broth (page 119)

1 cup de-stemmed and chopped kale

¼ cup chopped fresh cilantro

Ayurvedic Kichadi

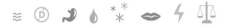

Many years ago, I spent some time in India and regularly ate homemade kichadi, a comforting dish that really helped me when I felt sick. Kichadi is an ancient Indian dish that is synonymous with healing. It's meant to rebalance the body by supporting digestion and stimulating digestive fire. The recipe below is our take on it, but it still captures the essence of this restorative meal. It cooks into a soothing, warm stew that stimulates appetite and eases the stomach, mainly because of the spices. This is one of the best mains to eat wherever you are on your cancer journey; it can ease most side effects as well as reinvigorate your body and spirit. **SG**

1. Soak the mung beans in a bowl of room-temperature water for 8 hours before preparing. Use enough water so that the beans are covered. After they have soaked, drain and set aside.

2. Place a large pot or Dutch oven over medium heat and add the ghee. Once the ghee is hot, stir in the bay leaves, turmeric, cumin seeds, coriander, and salt and toast for 1–2 minutes. You'll know the spices are toasted when you start to smell them and some of them pop.

3. Add the onions and ginger, and sauté in the spices for 5 minutes.

4. Add the mung beans, rice, carrots, celery, squash, and water or Phyto Broth and stir to combine everything. Bring to a boil and then reduce to a simmer. Cover and simmer for 1 hour on low heat. Don't stir the pot again until after an hour.

5. After 1 hour, stir in the kale and allow it to steam in the hot kichadi. It will cook quickly, within 2 minutes.

6. Top your bowl of kichadi with cilantro.

7. You can store this in the fridge for up to 4 days or in the freezer for 4–5 months.

---

1 medium sweet potato, peeled

½ cup fresh parsley, finely
chopped

¼ cup diced red onion

1 garlic clove, minced

15 oz can chickpeas, drained
and rinsed, or 1½ cups
cooked chickpeas

⅓ cup chickpea flour

3 Tbsp tahini

2 Tbsp fresh lemon juice

½ tsp cumin

½ tsp sea salt

Pinch of pepper

¼ cup sesame seeds

1 Tbsp extra-virgin olive oil

Extra Boosts and Pairings:
Sunflower Hummus (page 206)

Quinoa Tabouli (page 185)

Turnip Beet Mash (page 197)

2 Tbsp coarsely chopped fresh
parsley

½ tsp sesame seeds

1 tsp za'atar

1 tsp tahini

Easy Falafels

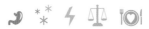

Falafels are the ultimate Middle Eastern street food, but we've given them a slight facelift: they're baked, rather than deep-fried, and we use our secret weapon ingredient—sweet potato. The result is a subtly sweet, zesty, and savory ball with punchy flavor and a great light texture. This recipe is a fan favorite among our clients, which is how we know you will love it too. Take these falafels with you wherever you go. They travel well, are freezer friendly, and make a perfect snack or meal, especially on days you have treatment. Load them in a pita or romaine leaf with a scoop of Sunflower Hummus and Quinoa Tabouli and voilà.

1. Preheat the oven to 375°F and line a baking sheet with parchment paper.
2. Use the S blade of a food processor to pulse the sweet potato, parsley, onions, and garlic together. Once a crumbly texture forms, add the chickpeas and pulse until they're distributed throughout the mixture but are still slightly intact. You don't want a creamy consistency.
3. Transfer the mixture to a big bowl and stir in the chickpea flour, tahini, lemon juice, cumin, salt, and pepper.
4. Take 2 heaping tablespoons of the mixture, form into a ball, and place it on the baking sheet. Repeat with the remaining mixture. You should end up with approximately 20 falafels.
5. Sprinkle sesame seeds over the falafels, then lightly drizzle olive oil over all of them. Bake in the oven for 25–30 minutes; no flipping necessary.
6. Eat the falafels as part of a salad, or in whole-grain pitas, or on a bed of roasted vegetables. Sprinkle parsley, sesame seeds, and za'atar, and then drizzle tahini over top for a full-on Middle Eastern experience.
7. Store in an airtight container in the fridge for up to 5 days or in the freezer for up to 2 months.

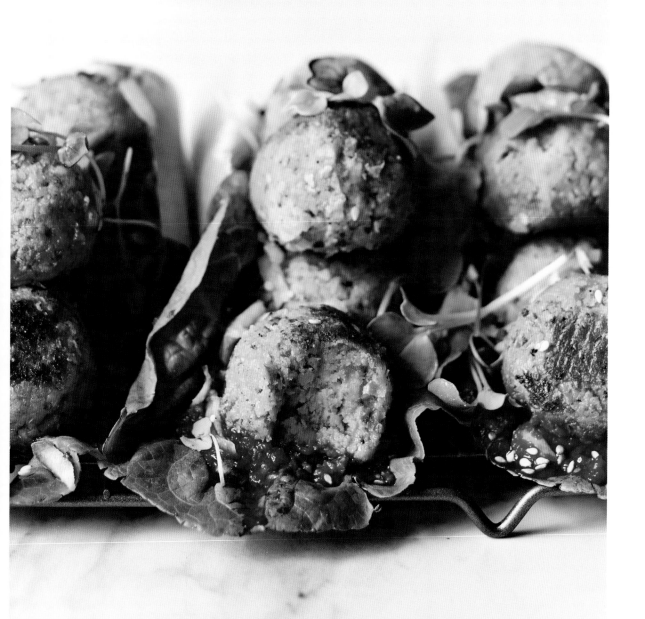

We like pairing the falafels with our Turnip Beet Mash (page 197). It's delicious.

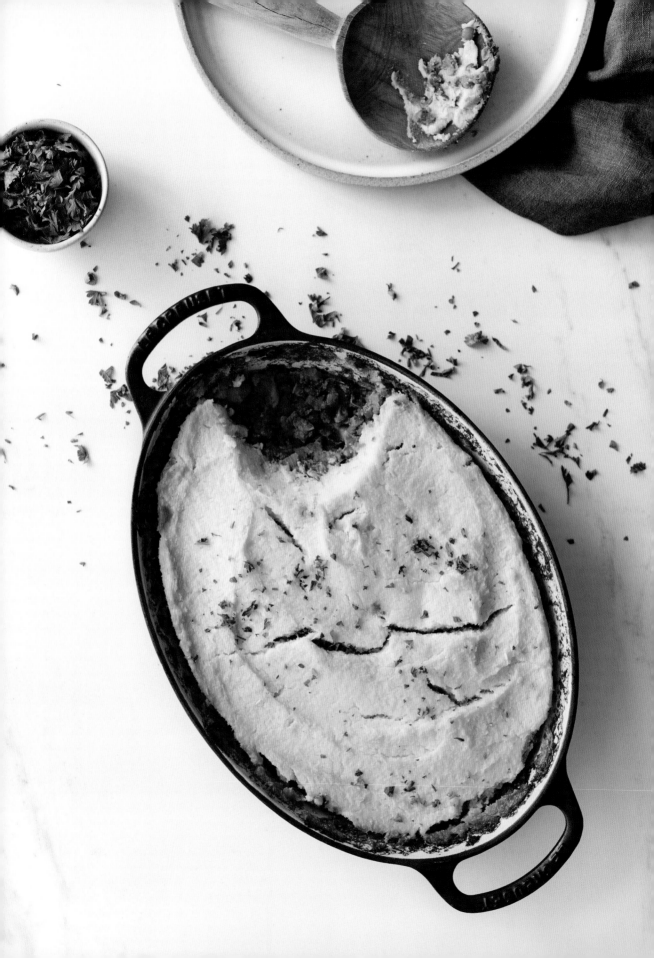

Topping:

1 head cauliflower, chopped
into florets

2 parsnips, peeled and diced

2 Tbsp ghee, butter, or extra-
virgin olive oil

½ tsp sea salt

Pinch of pepper

Filling:

1 Tbsp ghee or extra-virgin olive
oil

1 small yellow onion, diced

2 cloves garlic, chopped

2 carrots, peeled and diced

½ cup coarsely chopped
shiitake mushrooms

2 celery stalks, diced

½ tsp dried thyme or 1 tsp fresh
thyme leaves

½ tsp sea salt

Pinch of pepper

1 cup dried green lentils

2 cups Phyto Broth (page 119)
or store-bought organic
vegetable broth

3 Tbsp chopped fresh parsley

Lentil Shepherd's Pie

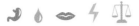

This is not your average shepherd's pie. We use parsnips and cauliflower as the topping instead of white potatoes, and we also use potent immune-enhancing ingredients like shiitake mushrooms, garlic, our Phyto Broth, and high-fiber, protein-rich lentils. Make this dish when you have energy, then freeze it and reheat when you need a quick meal.

1. To make the topping, put the cauliflower and parsnips in a pot with ½ cup of water. Turn the heat to medium, cover the pot, and let simmer for 10–12 minutes, or until soft.

2. Place the steamed cauliflower and parsnips (along with any water that's left in the pot), ghee, salt, and pepper in a food processor and blend until creamy. Alternatively, if you're making this by hand, mash with a potato masher and mix together.

3. To make the filling, place a large pot on the stove over medium heat. Add the ghee, onions, garlic, carrots, mushrooms, and celery. Sauté for 3 minutes, or until the onions are translucent, and then add the thyme, salt, and pepper.

4. Add the lentils to the pot, cover with broth, and bring to a boil. Then reduce the heat, cover, and simmer for 30 minutes. The lentils will be cooked through, and the liquid will be absorbed. Then stir in the fresh parsley.

5. Preheat the oven to 375°F and line a casserole dish with parchment paper. Spoon in the lentil filling and spread it evenly along the bottom of the dish, then top with the mashed cauliflower mixture. Flatten it with a spoon, making sure to spread the lentil filling to the edges of the dish.

6. Bake in the oven for 30 minutes, broiling for 3 minutes at the end so that the topping is set and lightly browned. You can keep in the fridge for 4 days or freeze leftover pie for 3–4 months. It's best to cut the pie and freeze it as individual portions for easy and quick reheating.

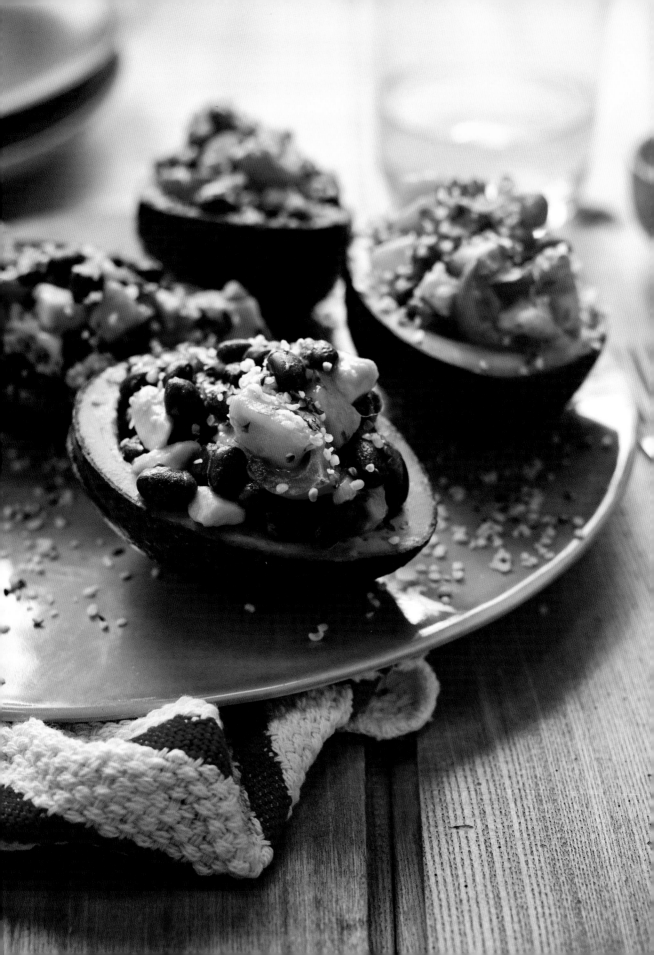

———————

1 mango

15 oz can black beans, or
1 cup cooked black beans

1 lime, juiced

½ red pepper, diced

¼ cup fresh cilantro, finely
chopped

1 Tbsp extra-virgin olive oil

¼ tsp cumin

¼ tsp sea salt

Pinch of pepper

2 ripe avocados

Extra Boosts:

1 Tbsp hemp seeds

½ cup broccoli, sunflower,
or pea sprouts

Salsa-Stuffed Avocado

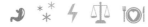

We've been stuffing squash and red pepper for years; now it's avocado's turn. It's only natural that we paired a ripe avocado with a zesty, fresh black bean and mango salsa that's got a real Tex Mex kick. The salsa gets heaped into the avocado (no cooking and little cleanup—hooray!), and with a nice garnish of cilantro, it's ready to eat. This is one of our quickest recipes, and it's excellent to eat before or between treatments, since the fat and fiber content are so high and it helps strengthen the body. You can eat half the avocado or a full one; either way, we recommend eating this with a big spoon.

1. Cut the mango into cubes by first slicing the mango lengthwise on either side of the pit. (The pit lies right in the center of the mango; you don't actually remove it; rather, cut around it.) Score each mango half into small cubes, and then scoop the cubes out with a spoon, being careful when scoring to not cut yourself.

2. Place the mango cubes in a bowl, and add the black beans, lime juice, red pepper, cilantro, olive oil, cumin, salt, and pepper to the bowl. Toss everything together.

3. Slice the two avocados in half, and then remove the pit and score the avocado halves as you did the mango. Scoop out a few of the cubes from the middle to create a well in the center. You can add those cubes to the salsa or eat them while preparing this.

4. Spoon the salsa into the wells of the avocados, and enjoy right away.

If you aren't going to eat this recipe right away, the salsa will last in an airtight container in the fridge for up to 5 days. We recommend waiting to cut the avocado until you are ready to eat.

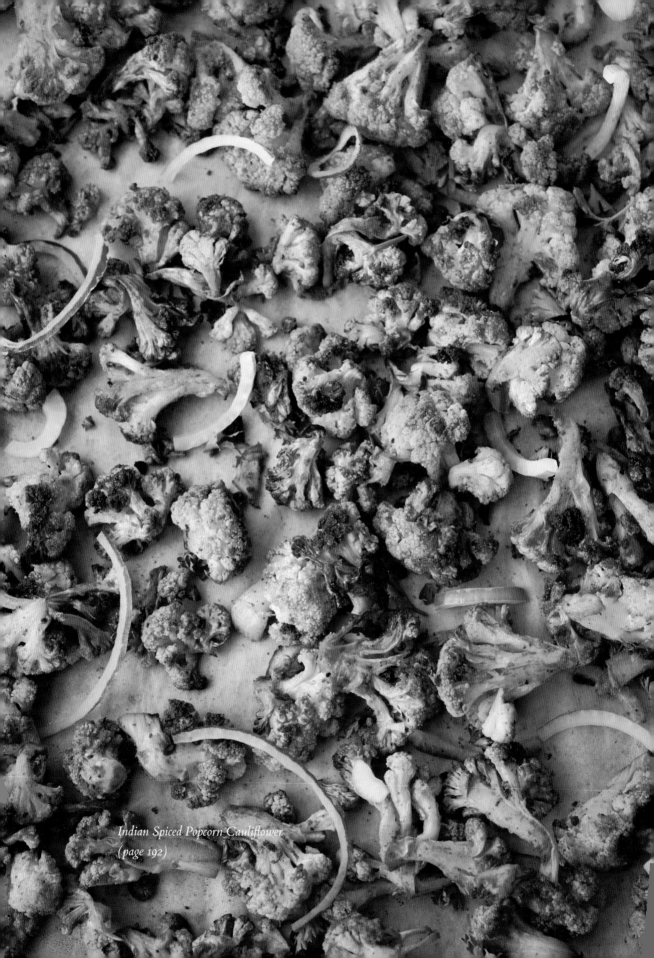

Indian Spiced Popcorn Cauliflower
(page 192)

SIDES

Side dishes are where many of our vegetable recipes live. It's in this section that you'll find creative and unique ways of preparing veggies and grains. We've mentioned many times before that digestion starts with your eyes, so the plate or bowl in front of you better look appetizing! That's why our goal is to create beautiful (and tasty) side dishes with a rainbow of colors that will stimulate your appetite and provide your body with an array of phytonutrients to keep you strong and healthy.

Prep Tips for Side Dishes

These are our tried-and-true tips for making prepping *easy*. Opening your fridge door and seeing shelves lined with chopped colorful vegetables and cooked grains and proteins is one of the best feelings. It means that putting together a meal will be easy, with no extra work and no mess. It's like having your own salad bar right in your fridge.

- If you have the energy, we recommend washing, chopping, and then storing a variety of vegetables in the fridge, as well as cooking ½–1 cup's worth of grains like quinoa, rice, and millet.

- If your body can't tolerate raw vegetables, lightly sauté or steam your veggies of choice to make them more digestible and easier to eat. There is no need to skip veggies altogether; your body needs them during treatment.

- Most raw veggies can last up to two weeks, but it's best to use them up as quickly as you can to maintain their nutrients. Cooked grains last up to four days in the fridge, but they can also be frozen for two to three months. Marinades, sauces, and dressings last 4–7 days in the fridge.

- Keep a variety of containers and jars on hand to store your prep. We prefer large ziplock bags and glass containers with lids that snap and lock to maintain freshness.

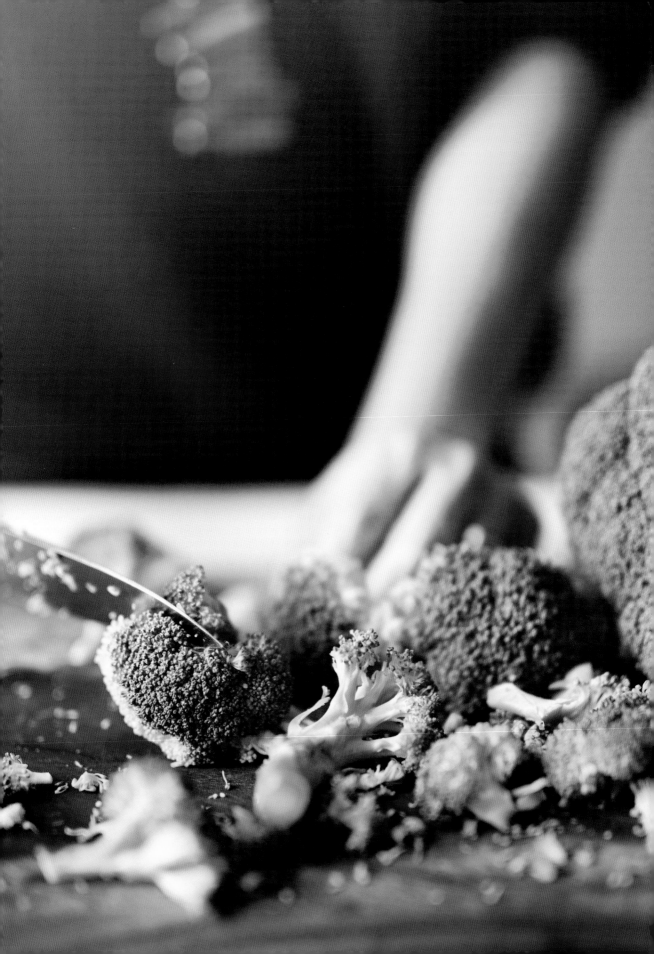

½ cup dried arame

2 tsp virgin coconut oil

½ cup diced yellow onion

1 Tbsp grated peeled ginger root

3 carrots, peeled and sliced into matchsticks

4 cups de-stemmed and chopped kale

2 tsp tamari

2 tsp toasted sesame oil

2 Tbsp sesame seeds or hemp seeds

NUTRITION NOTE Arame is rich in an array of minerals like iodine, iron, magnesium, and zinc. Most sea vegetables also contain antioxidant power through their vitamin and phyto-nutrient content to help protect your cells. Seaweeds also contain a significant amount of protein for a vegetable.

Toasted Sesame Arame and Carrot Kale Sauté

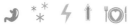

You'd be surprised how many people think seaweed is just plain weird. You may be one of those people, but I promise that after the first bite of this dish, you won't think it's weird anymore. I created this recipe for a seaweed-hungry client who wanted all the health benefits of this sea vegetable (most notably, its link with slowing cancer cell growth) without the typical pungent flavor. Tender sweet onions, a kick of ginger, and the familiar taste of carrots and kale are the perfect match with savory arame, which will taste a lot less like the ocean than other varieties of seaweeds. **SG**

1. Soak the arame in a bowl of warm water for 15 minutes. The arame should be fully submerged as it softens and expands.
2. In the meantime, put a pan over medium heat. Add 2 teaspoons of coconut oil and sauté the onions and ginger for 5 minutes.
3. Add the carrots to the pan and cook for 5 more minutes, or until they begin to soften.
4. Drain the arame and throw it into the pan along with the kale. Stir in the tamari and toasted sesame oil. Sauté for 3 minutes, or until the kale is cooked.
5. Top with sesame seeds or hemp seeds.
6. You can store leftovers in the fridge for 3–4 days. We think this dish tastes best when warm, so you can reheat it again in a small pan (but you can always try eating it cold).

You can find arame at health food stores or online.

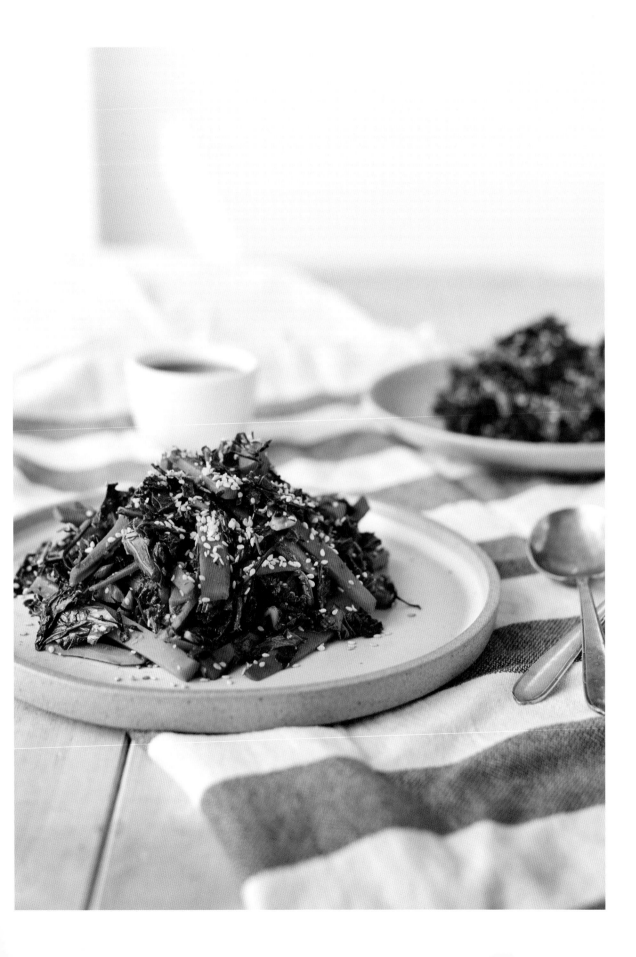

Tamari Roasted Brussels Sprouts

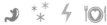

2 lbs Brussels sprouts, bottoms
   cut off, halved

1½ cups thinly sliced red onion
   (about ½ onion)

2 Tbsp extra-virgin olive oil

1 Tbsp tamari

1 Tbsp pure maple syrup

¼ cup fresh cilantro, parsley, or
   a combination

Extra Boost:

2 tsp hemp seeds

When most people think of Brussels sprouts, a big bowl of steamed Brussels sprouts probably comes to mind. Well, Brussels sprouts have come a long way, baby, and they're no longer that unappetizing vegetable that people love to hate. I never really ate Brussels sprouts growing up, so when I was given a bag of them, I wasn't sure what to do with them. So, like any good cook, I smothered them in maple syrup and tamari, and a wildly satisfying dish was born. If you are a lover of sweet and savory, this recipe will please, especially if your taste buds have altered. **TG**

1. Preheat the oven to 375°F and line a baking sheet with parchment paper.
2. Spread the Brussels sprouts and onions on the baking sheet.
3. Pour the oil, tamari, and maple syrup over the veggies and mix well so they are coated.
4. Roast for 30 minutes, or until the onions are soft and the Brussels sprouts have browned, shrunk, and crisped on the outside. Top with the fresh cilantro and/or parsley right before eating. You can also add hemp seeds if you like.

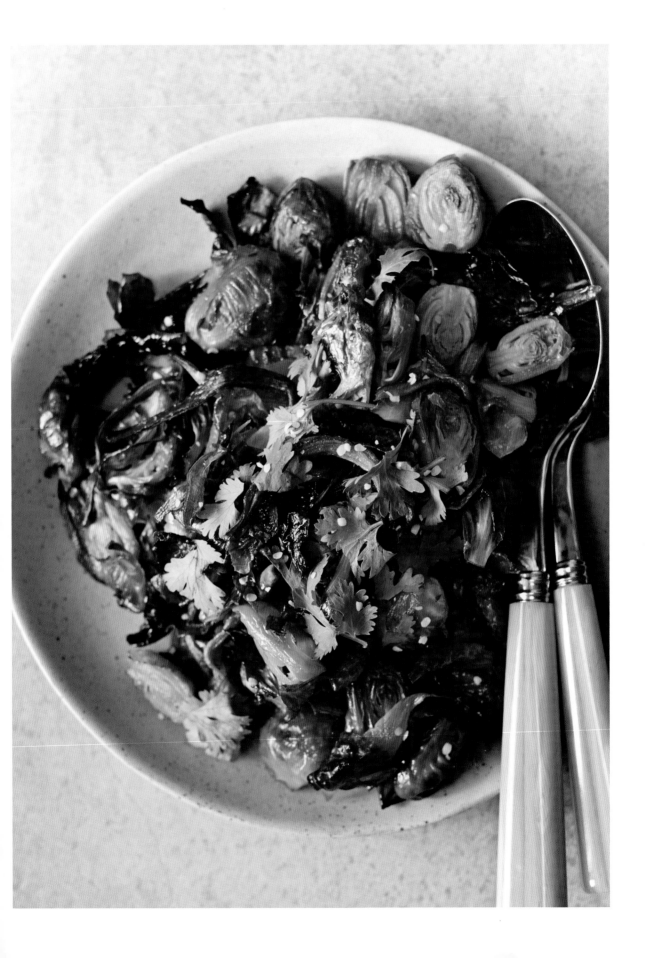

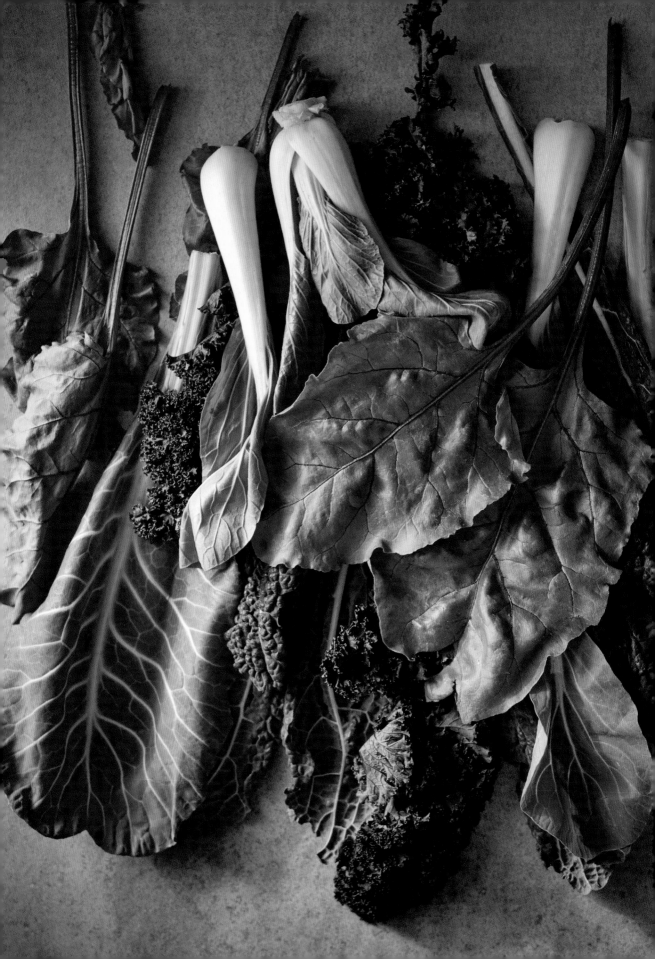

1 Tbsp virgin coconut oil or ghee

2 cloves garlic, minced

1 inch ginger root, peeled and minced

2 cups de-stemmed and chopped kale

1 cup de-stemmed and chopped collards

1 cup chopped dandelion or mustard greens (or substitute more collards)

¼ cup Organic Chicken, Phyto, or Strong Bones Broth (pages 118–120), or store-bought organic broth

¼ tsp sea salt

Pinch of pepper

Golden Turmeric Sauce (page 247)

NUTRITION NOTE Leafy greens are packed with vitamin C, vitamin A, vitamin K, B vitamins, calcium, fiber, and phytonutrients like sulforaphane and indoles, which support the liver in neutralizing toxins and chemicals and excreting them from the body.

Emerald-Green Garlic Sauté

Leafy greens are nature's superfood, and the ones we chose for this recipe are extra super. Their slightly bitter flavor (which we offset with the subtly sweet coconut oil) will help stimulate your appetite during treatment. Garlic and ginger warm up the dish and boost its nutrition and flavor, which is just so much better than a plate of plain steamed veggies. Our Golden Turmeric Sauce is a medley of creamy, earthy tahini with hints of lemon, the subtle bite of garlic, and the heat of ginger that will make any vegetable taste divine!

1. In a wide saucepan, heat the coconut oil and then add the garlic and ginger. Sauté for 30 seconds, or until fragrant.

2. Mix in the kale, collards, and dandelion so that they are coated in the oil, garlic, and ginger. Pour in the broth, cover the pan, and simmer on low for 3–4 minutes, or until the greens are bright green and tender. Season with salt and pepper.

3. Make the Golden Turmeric Sauce. Smother the greens in the golden sauce or serve it on the side as a dipping sauce.

4. The cooked greens can be stored in the fridge, in an airtight container, for 4 days. The sauce can also be stored in an airtight container in the fridge for up to 5 days.

If you're tired or short on time, you can skip the step of simmering the greens in broth. They'll still be absolutely delicious without it! You can also skip the Golden Turmeric Sauce or serve this with another sauce that you like (check out all of our sauces, starting on page 241).

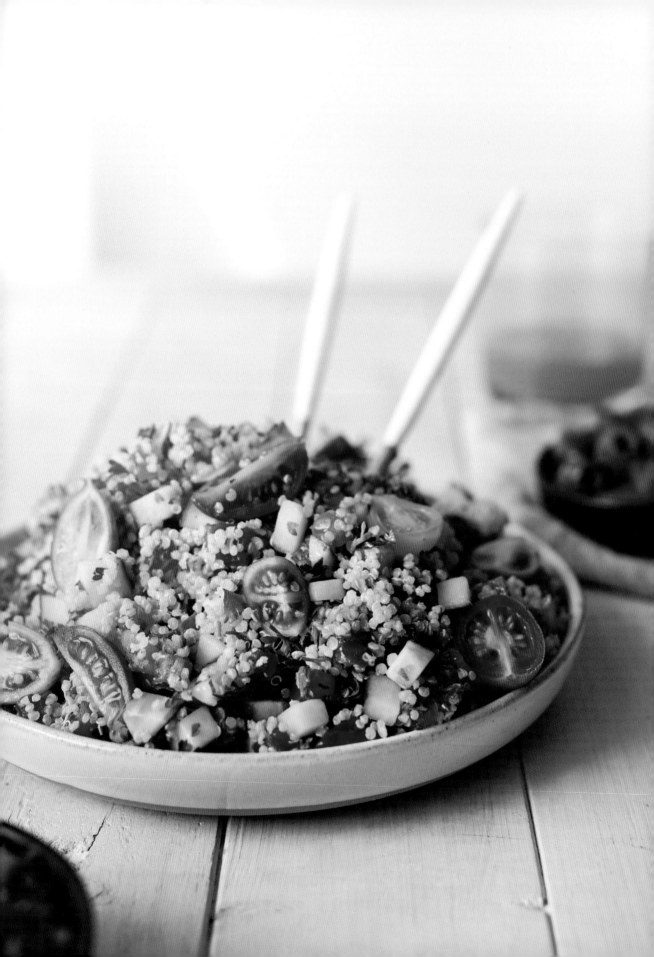

MAKES 4 SERVINGS

PREP TIME: 15 MINUTES

COOK TIME: 15 MINUTES

½ cup quinoa

1 cup water

2 cups finely chopped flat-leaf
parsley

½ cup finely chopped fresh
mint

1 cup halved cherry tomatoes

1 cup finely diced cucumber

¼ cup fresh lemon juice

2 Tbsp extra-virgin olive oil

½ tsp sea salt

Pinch of pepper

Tahini Lemon Zest Dressing
(page 251)

NUTRITION NOTE The fresh
herbs in this recipe will give
your immune system extra support, and they'll help digestion.
Parsley contains antioxidants
that protect your cells from
carcinogens.

Quinoa Tabouli

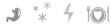

Our favorite Middle Eastern restaurant in Toronto serves up
the most delicious hummus and salad, embellished with tart
pomegranate and aromatic za'atar. As a result, we are always
coming up with ways to use more tahini (which we have a
mild obsession with), lemon, and fresh herbs in our recipes.
Naturally, we came up with our own version of tabouli, a
classic dish made with earthy parsley, refreshing mint, and
chewy bulgur wheat. In ours, we've swapped out the bulgur
for nutty-tasting quinoa to add extra protein and make it
gluten-free.

1. In a small pot, combine the quinoa and water. Bring to a
   boil and then reduce the heat to low. Cover and simmer for
   15 minutes.
2. Meanwhile, toss the parsley, mint, tomatoes, and cucumber
   in a large bowl.
3. Once the quinoa is cooked, it should be fluffy and all the
   water will be absorbed. Take it off the heat and let it cool.
   You can put it in the fridge for 5 minutes to cool it down
   quickly.
4. Toss the quinoa with the vegetables, lemon juice, olive oil,
   salt, and pepper.
5. Drizzle 2–4 tablespoons of the Tahini Lemon Zest Dressing
   over each serving, or more if you prefer.
6. The leftovers will keep in an airtight container in the fridge
   for up to 4 days.

Flat-leaf parsley has more flavor than curly parsley. But if you aren't able
to find flat-leaf, then you can sub in curly leaf.

You can use a food processor to chop all the veggies if you're low on
energy and want to save time.

Loaded Vegetable Salad

2 cups de-stemmed and finely
chopped kale

1½ cups sliced cucumber

1 cup thinly sliced purple
cabbage

½ cup thinly sliced radishes
(about 4 radishes)

½ cup diced red pepper
(1 small red pepper)

1 carrot, peeled and julienned

½ avocado, diced

¼ cup chopped flat-leaf parsley

Toppings:
¼ cup broccoli sprouts

1 Tbsp raw sunflower seeds

1 Tbsp raw pumpkin seeds

1 Tbsp hemp seeds

Sunflower Seed "Caesar"
Dressing (page 248)

We love a salad that has it all: loud colors, crunchy, soft, and juicy textures, and punchy, zippy, and sweet flavors. The Loaded Vegetable Salad is meant to be a "use it all up" salad, meaning whatever you've got in the fridge, throw it in! You can use this recipe as the base and add whatever you want, or just follow the recipe as is, because it's a good one. This is a filling salad since the vegetables are all bursting with fiber. You can make this into a meal by topping it with one of our meat or veggie burgers found in our omnivore mains or vegetarian mains recipe sections.

1. Toss all the chopped vegetables together in a big bowl.
2. Make the salad dressing in a separate jar.
3. Top the portion of salad you are eating immediately with the sprouts, seeds, and a drizzle of salad dressing, and enjoy.
4. Store leftover salad in an airtight container. It will keep in the fridge for up to 5 days.
5. Store the dressing in a glass jar and then dress salad when you're ready to eat it again.

Since this is a raw salad, it may be difficult to chew if your mouth is sensitive. A solution is to lightly steam the vegetables or add an extra helping of dressing to soften them up a bit.

We recommend only dressing the portion of salad you are going to eat right away. That way the rest of the salad will save better for other meals.

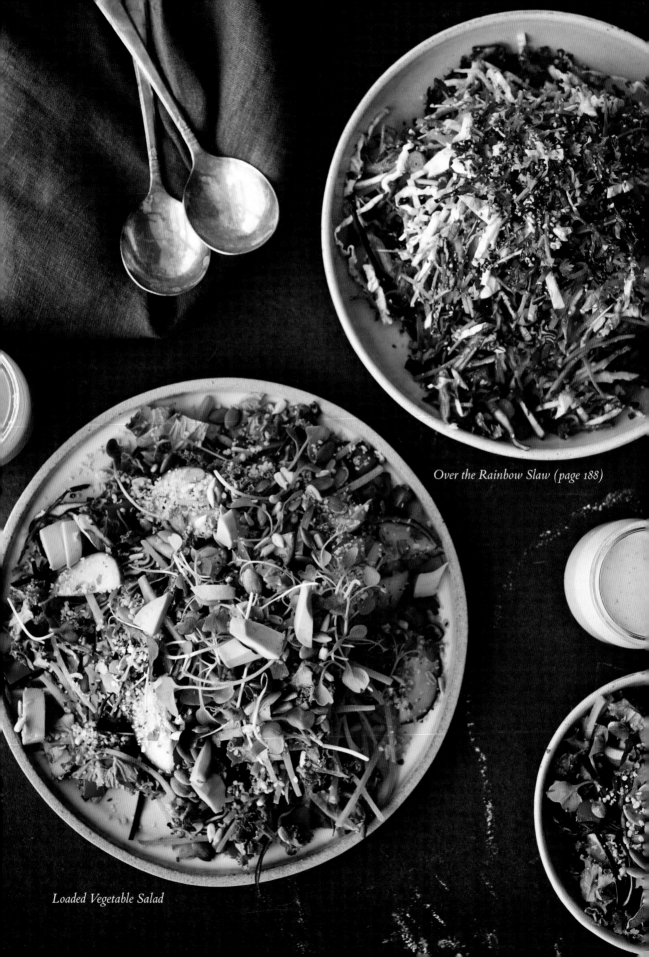

Over the Rainbow Slaw *(page 188)*

Loaded Vegetable Salad

---

1 medium beet, peeled

2 medium carrots, peeled

1 cup thinly sliced purple cabbage

1 cup thinly sliced savoy or napa cabbage

1 cup thinly sliced green or purple cabbage

½ cup chopped fresh parsley

2 green onions, finely chopped

Flax Oil Anti-Inflammation Dressing (page 250)

Toppings:

3 Tbsp hemp seeds

1 Tbsp chia seeds

¼ cup sauerkraut

NUTRITION NOTE Cabbage is a cruciferous veggie that supports the blood and immune system, and helps with detoxification. Cruciferous veggies are one of the most important foods to eat for cancer prevention and recovery.

Over the Rainbow Slaw

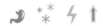

For those of you who think you're not a fan of cabbage: this salad will make you one with its refreshing and energizing bite. Savoy and napa cabbage are both softer and milder than the sturdy, crisp purple and green cabbages, so pairing them makes for a beautiful rainbow of colors that's full of texture. And, the sweet taste of beets and carrots helps balance the bitterness of the crunchy cabbage. Once you let the cabbage marinate in the dressing, it softens a bit, becoming easier to chew and more flavorful too.

1. If you have a food processor, use the grating attachment to grate the beet and carrots. Use the slicing attachment to slice the cabbages. Otherwise, grate the beet and carrots by hand and slice the cabbages with a knife as thinly as you can.

2. In a large bowl, combine the beet, carrots, cabbage, parsley, and green onions.

3. Prepare the dressing and pour it over the serving of slaw you are going to eat. Keep the extra dressing in the fridge in an airtight jar to be used again later.

4. Top with hemp seeds, chia seeds, and sauerkraut.

5. If the slaw is undressed, you can keep it in the refrigerator for 5 days. If it's dressed, it's best to eat it within 2 days.

If you can't digest raw cabbage, lightly steam or sauté it in some coconut oil before mixing it with the other veggies. Also, the more finely you can slice the cabbage, the easier it is to chew. A mandoline or food processor with a slicer attachment are both really helpful here.

MAKES 4 SERVINGS

PREP TIME: 10 MINUTES

COOK TIME: 35–40 MINUTES

Sweet potato mash:

1 tsp + 1 Tbsp ghee or virgin coconut oil

3 cloves garlic, chopped

4 cups cubed peeled sweet potato (leave the peel on if organic)

¼ tsp sea salt

Pinch of pepper

Sautéed mushrooms:

1 Tbsp ghee

4 cups mixed mushrooms, like shiitake and cremini, de-stemmed and chopped

1 tsp dried thyme or 4 tsp fresh thyme leaves

½ tsp sea salt

Pinch of pepper

Toppings:

2 tsp hemp seeds

2 tsp flax oil or extra-virgin olive oil

Sautéed Mushrooms over Sweet Potato Mash

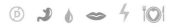

Get ready to eat some magic mushrooms! No, not those kind; this is a cookbook, come on! These mushrooms are magical thanks to the powerful medicinal properties they have that help protect your immune system. As you sauté them, the mushrooms gently caramelize to become sweet without the addition of sugar (just another one of their magic tricks!). They get served on buttery mashed sweet potatoes that have been blended with an ample amount of sautéed garlic and ghee. Together the mushrooms and sweet potatoes perfectly complement each other's earthy and sweet tones. A pleasing dish to stimulate an appetite.

1. To make the sweet potato mash, set a pot over medium heat. Add 1 teaspoon of the ghee and sauté the garlic until fragrant, about 45 seconds.

2. Add the sweet potato, then pour in ¾ cup of water. Cover the pot and simmer for 15–20 minutes, or until the sweet potatoes are soft. Add the salt, pepper, and 1 tablespoon of ghee, and mash by hand or in the food processor until smooth.

3. Meanwhile, sauté the mushrooms. Place a pan on medium heat and add the ghee. Then add the mushrooms, thyme, salt, and pepper. Sauté, stirring frequently, until the water from the mushrooms evaporates, 7–10 minutes.

4. Spoon the mushrooms on top of the mashed sweet potatoes and top with hemp seeds and a drizzle of flax oil. If you will be reheating this dish later, wait to add the flax oil until it's been reheated, to prevent damaging the oil.

5. Store in an airtight container in the fridge for up to 5 days.

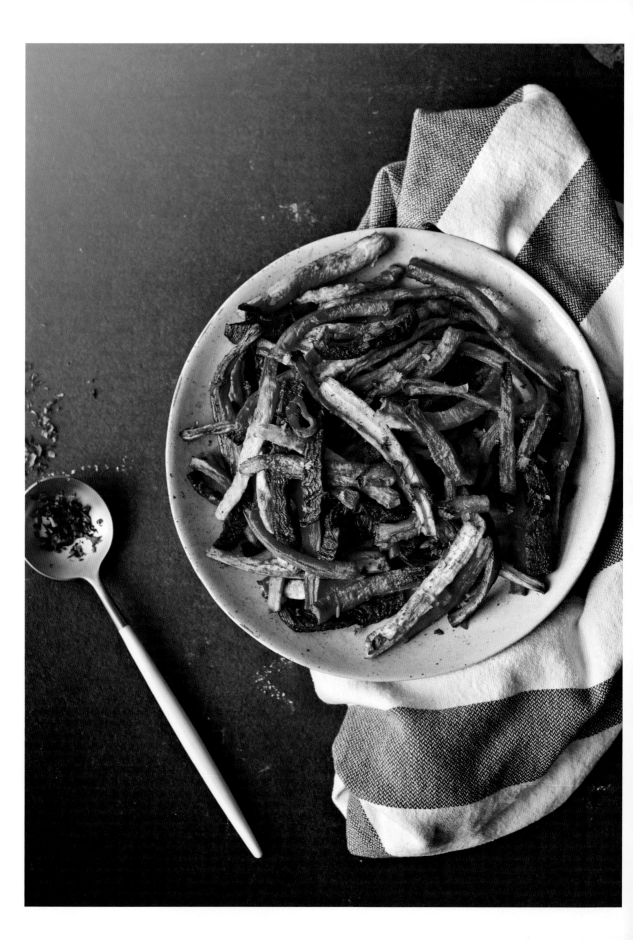

———————

2 parsnips, peeled

2 carrots, peeled

1 beet, peeled

½ daikon radish, peeled

2 Tbsp extra-virgin olive oil

1 tsp granulated garlic powder

½ tsp sea salt

Pinch of pepper

Topping:
1–2 Tbsp fresh parsley,
    chopped

Colorful Root Fries

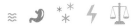

It's hard to imagine that fries made with root veggies other than potatoes can be just as good (or better!) than their cousin, the french fry. Using a combo of veggies with varying colors means greater protection of your health and a whackload more flavor. We have a culinary secret for you: granulated garlic is the key to making baked fries awesome. Do not skimp on this seasoning when you're making this recipe. It brings out the flavor of the veggies, adds its own *je ne sais quoi*, and infuses a good smack of garlic into each fry.

1. Preheat the oven to 375°F and line two baking sheets with parchment paper.
2. Slice the root veggies in half lengthwise, place the flat edge of the vegetable on your cutting board and cut lengthwise into thin fries. The daikon will require a few more slices to achieve the french fry shape.
3. Toss the fries with the olive oil, garlic powder, salt, and pepper and spread them out on the baking sheets. Don't overcrowd them, otherwise they will steam rather than crisp. Bake for 25–30 minutes, flipping them halfway through. Take them out when they have shrunken slightly and feel lightly crisp on the outside. Top with fresh parsley.

Daikon is a long, thick white cylindrical radish. It's typically pretty large, so you will probably only need to use half of one for this recipe. You can use the other half in salads, peel it into ribbons, spiralize it into noodles, or cut it into raw veggie sticks.

If you're strapped for time, cut the vegetables into thinner fries so that they cook faster.

1 large head of cauliflower or
2 small heads, chopped into
florets (about 6 cups)

3 Tbsp ghee or virgin coconut
oil, melted

2 tsp garam masala

1 tsp cumin

1 tsp ground ginger

1 tsp turmeric

¼–½ tsp sea salt

Pinch of pepper

Topping:
1–2 Tbsp fresh parsley or
cilantro, chopped

NUTRITION NOTE Cauli-
flower contains sulforaphane,
a compound that studies have
found can help kill cancer cells.
Turmeric slows down the spread
of cancer and has been shown
to make chemotherapy more
effective.

Indian Spiced Popcorn Cauliflower

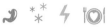

I was standing in my kitchen with Jess, one of our recipe testers, both of us staring at the timer, waiting patiently for the fragrant cauliflower to be crisp enough to take out of the oven. With each recipe we tested during the course of writing this book, we always promised to save some for our friends and family to try so they could tell us what they thought. We excitedly huddled over the tray of golden-stained cauliflower on the stove top. And almost as quickly as we took the first bite, the tray was empty—the phytonutrient-rich cauliflower was so addictively crispy, tender, and perfect that we had eaten every last piece. We looked at each other, slightly embarrassed that there would be no leftovers to share. So we made another batch—and then ate that one too. That's how I know you will love this recipe, and remember, sharing is optional. **TG**

1. Preheat the oven to 350°F and line two baking sheets with parchment paper.
2. Place the cauliflower on the baking sheets. The smaller you chop the florets, the faster this dish will roast. Don't overcrowd the cauliflower or it won't crisp up.
3. Pour the ghee over the cauliflower, and then sprinkle the spices over top. Mix with your hands or a spoon to make sure the cauliflower is well coated.
4. Roast in the oven for 30–35 minutes, or until slightly crisp and golden. Top with fresh parsley or cilantro.
5. Store in an airtight container in the fridge for up to a week.

If you're not a fan of these spices, roast the cauliflower with just salt and pepper, and it will be equally delicious and addictive.

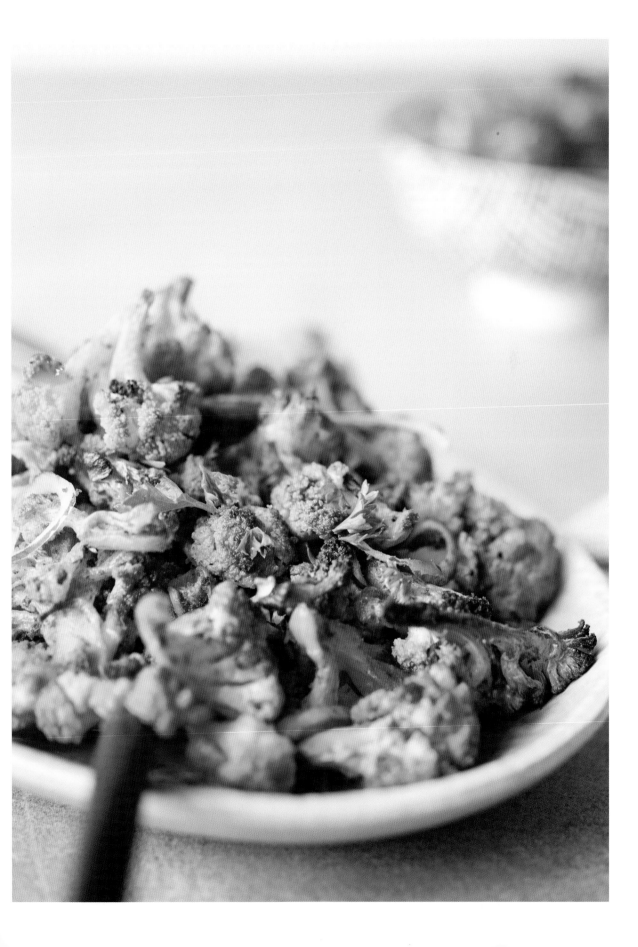

---

3 Tbsp ghee, butter, or extra-virgin olive oil

3 cloves garlic, minced

1 bunch rapini, chopped (5 loosely packed cups)

¼ tsp sea salt

Pinch of pepper

½ cup raw walnuts, coarsely chopped

¼ cup sundried tomatoes, sliced

¼ cup kalamata olives, pitted and sliced

NUTRITION NOTE Rapini is part of the cruciferous family, which makes it rich in phytonutrients that help your liver detoxify carcinogens out of the body. The olives in this recipe add a salty flavor with the benefit of fiber, healthy fat, and vitamin E, an antioxidant that protects cells from mutation.

Garlic Rapini with Sundried Tomatoes

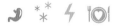

When I was a kid, I always looked forward to the evenings when my mom stopped at the local Italian restaurant and picked up food to go so we'd have an easy but completely satisfying dinner. It was the only time that I ever remember eating rapini, or broccoli rabe as we called it, that didn't taste bitter. The secret, I discovered, was garlic. Not just a little clove of garlic, but so much that the greens were smothered in the pure deliciousness of sweet, mouthwatering minced garlic sautéed in olive oil. We made this Living Kitchen recipe in the hope of winning our clients over with rapini, and the fresh-pressed garlic does the trick every time. If you've been skeptical of rapini, please do give this version a try! **SG**

1. Place a large pan over medium heat and add the ghee along with the garlic. Sauté until the garlic is fragrant, about 45 seconds. Then add the rapini, salt, and pepper. Sauté for 7–10 minutes, or until the rapini is wilted and soft.

2. In the meantime, lightly toast the walnuts in the oven on a small baking sheet for 4 minutes at 375°F. We recommend roasting nuts in the oven instead of on the stove top because it ensures the heat is well dispersed and the nuts are less likely to burn.

3. Remove the rapini from the heat and top with toasted walnuts, sundried tomatoes, and olives. Drizzle some extra-virgin olive oil over top before serving to increase your intake of nutritious fat.

Rapini cooks down a lot. It will look like a lot when you chop up the fresh bunch of leaves, but when cooked, it will reduce in bulk significantly.

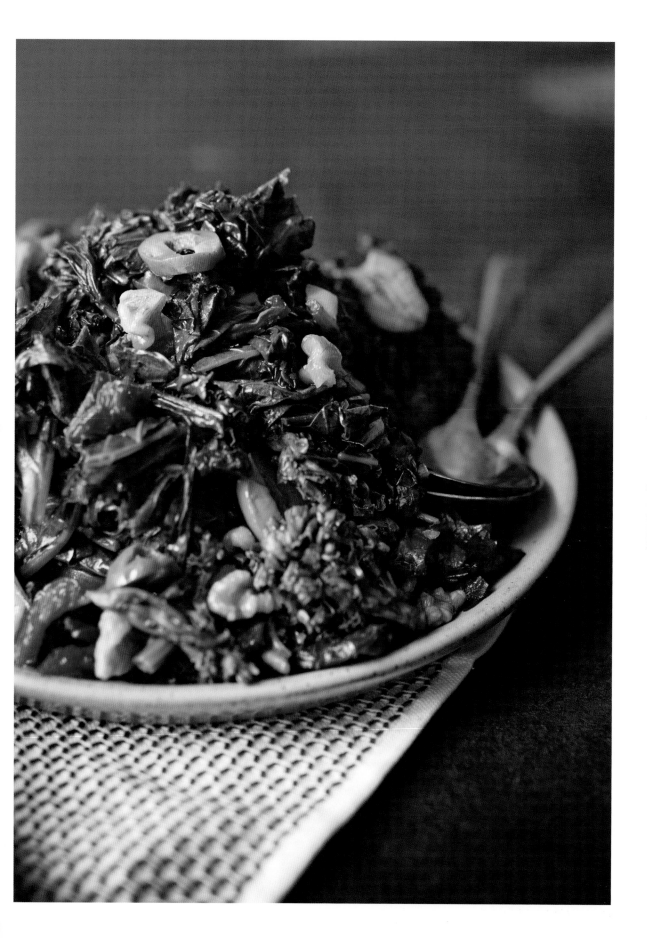

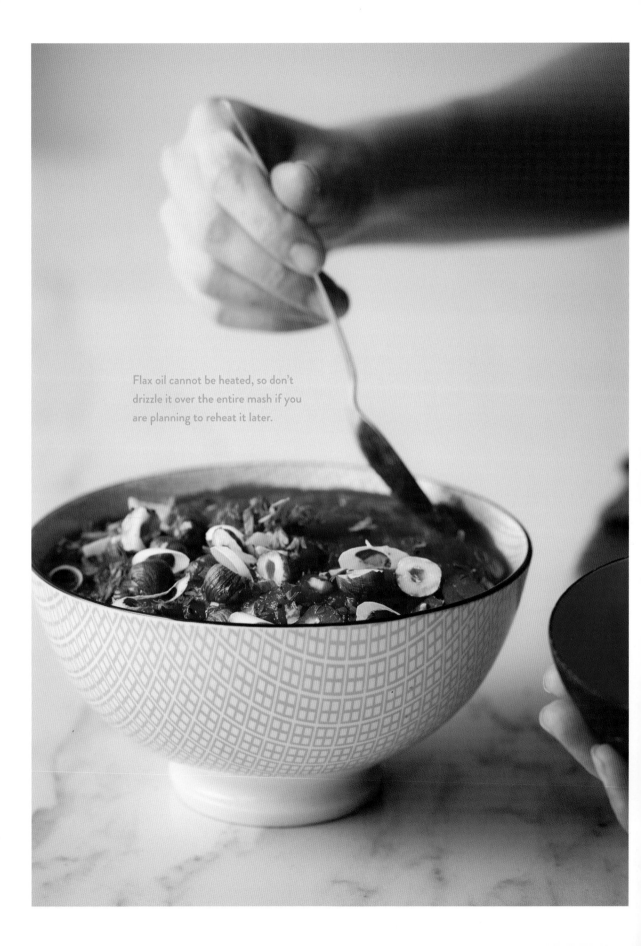

Flax oil cannot be heated, so don't
drizzle it over the entire mash if you
are planning to reheat it later.

———————

Roasted garlic:

1 bulb of garlic

1 tsp extra-virgin olive oil

Pinch each of sea salt and
 pepper

Mash:

1 cup coarsely chopped peeled
 beets (about 1 medium beet)

2 cups coarsely chopped
 peeled turnips (about 2 small
 turnips)

1⅓ cups coarsely chopped
 peeled parsnips (about 2
 medium parsnips)

2 Tbsp extra-virgin olive oil

¼ tsp sea salt

Pinch of pepper

2 tsp flax oil

Toppings:

¼ cup hazelnuts, halved

2 tsp chopped fresh parsley

1 green onion, sliced

Turnip Beet Mash

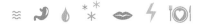

Bursting with purple hues, this creamy mash may just invigorate you from the color alone. Beets sometimes get a bad rap for
being too "earthy," but when they are steamed with other root
veggies, like turnips and parsnips, the earthy tones miraculously
turn sweet. This mash is simple to prepare and just what you
need to eat if you're experiencing the most common treatment
side effects like nausea, low appetite, or an upset stomach. Plus,
it's robustly flavorful, thanks to the roasted garlic. Roasted
garlic really makes everything better, don't you agree?

1. To make the roasted garlic, preheat the oven to 350°F. Slice
   the top off the garlic, drizzle with the olive oil, sprinkle salt
   and pepper over it, and wrap in tinfoil. Roast in the oven
   for 30–35 minutes. Once cooked, set aside.

2. Meanwhile, place the beets in a pot and cover them with
   water, just enough so that they're still peeking through.
   Cover the pot, bring to a boil, and then turn the temperature to medium-low and simmer for 10 minutes.

3. After 10 minutes, add the turnips and parsnips, and simmer
   for another 15–20 minutes, or until all the vegetables are
   soft.

4. Pour the cooked veggies into a food processor with the
   water they were cooked in (the water has many of the
   nutrients that leached out of the veggies). The water will
   be hot, so please be careful during this step.

5. The garlic will be hot, so use a towel or a glove to turn the
   sliced side down and squeeze out the roasted garlic cloves
   into the food processor. Add the olive oil, salt, and pepper,
   and blend until creamy. If you don't have a food processor,
   mash everything together by hand with a potato masher.

6. Drizzle a little flax oil over each serving and add the hazelnut, parsley and green onion toppings if you'd like.

7. Store in an airtight container in the fridge for up to 5 days
   or in the freezer for up to 6 months.

———————

3 sweet potatoes, sliced into wedges (leave skin on if organic)

2 Tbsp extra-virgin olive oil

1 tsp granulated garlic powder

1 tsp paprika

½ tsp chili powder

½ tsp dried oregano

½ tsp sea salt

Pinch of pepper

Topping:
1 Tbsp chopped fresh cilantro

Spiced Sweet Potato Wedges

It's sometimes hard to think of sweet potato wedges as a healthy dish when they're most commonly enjoyed in a pub alongside a cold beer. But the truth is, sweet potatoes have a huge amount of antioxidant power, and when combined with Southwestern spices, they actually stimulate the appetite. These potatoes are spiced perfectly (trust us, we've made this recipe over and over until they were) and baked at the exact temperature to achieve a crispy exterior with a soft interior. Enjoy these wedges on their own as a snack, or pair them with any of our main dishes.

1. Preheat the oven to 375°F and line two baking sheets with parchment paper.

2. Slice sweet potatoes in half lengthwise. Slice those halves in half again, then slice those quarters in half again until you have 8 wedges per potato. If you are working with a long, large sweet potato, cut it in half crosswise first before cutting it into wedges.

3. Place the sweet potatoes on one of the lined baking sheets. Pour the oil over top, sprinkle all the seasonings over the potatoes, and mix really well with your hands until they're evenly coated. Divide wedges between both baking sheets: you want them spread out flat and not overcrowded or else they won't get crispy.

4. Bake in the oven for 35–40 minutes, flipping the wedges after 20 minutes to cook both sides evenly. They should be slightly browned, crisp on the outside, and soft in the middle. Top the wedges with cilantro. We like to make some guacamole to dip the sweet potato wedges in.

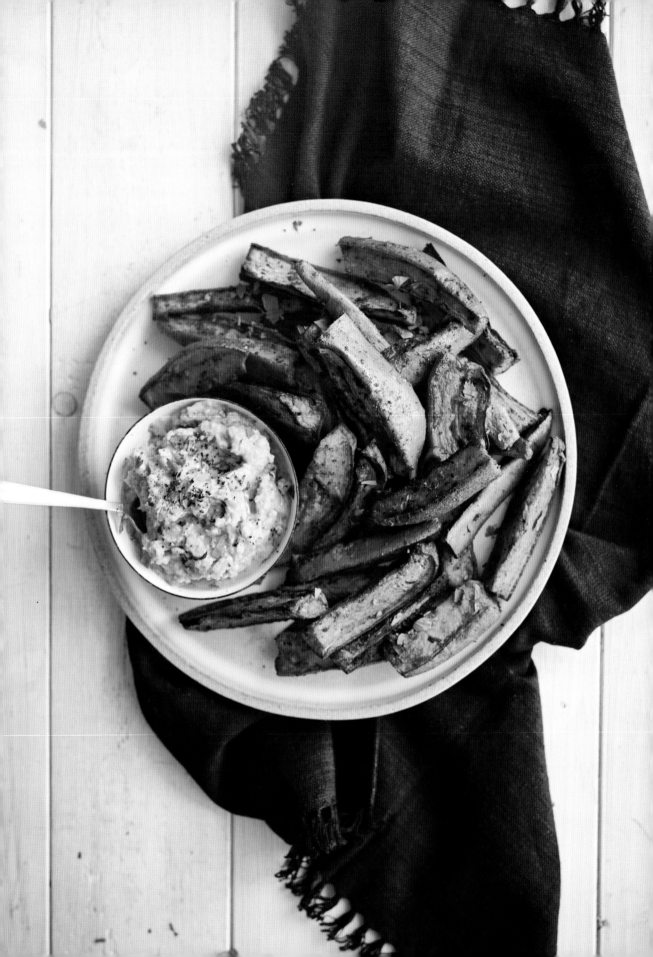

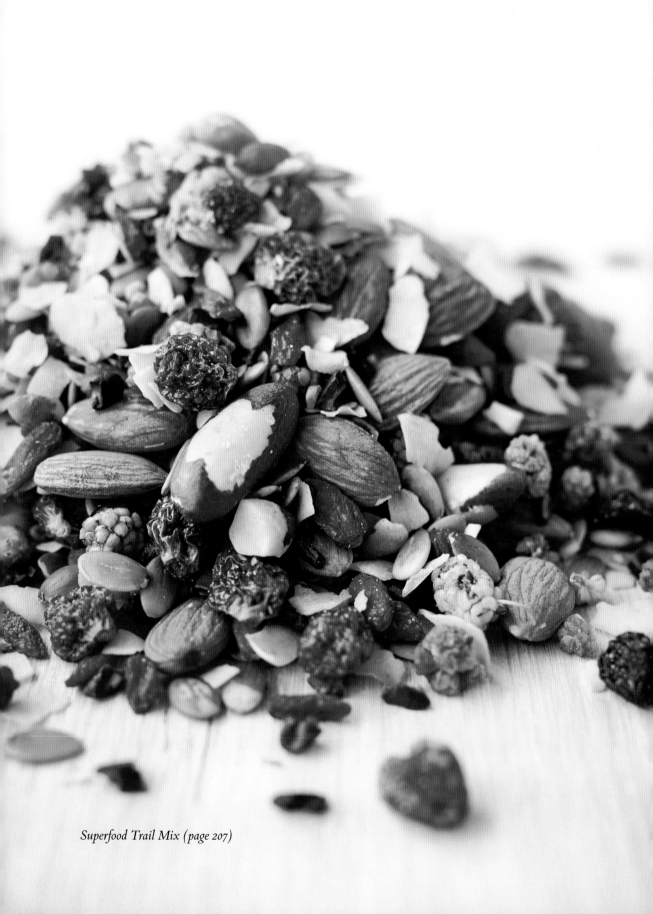

Superfood Trail Mix (page 207)

SNACKS

When you're undergoing treatment, there'll be times when you won't have a big appetite. That's where snacking can come in handy. It's a great way to get essential nutrients into your diet creatively, especially when eating is challenging for you. All of our snacks are easy to eat, great to take on the go, and promote strength and energy. Prepare a few of the recipes in this chapter each week so that you always have several quick, small snacks ready when you need them most.

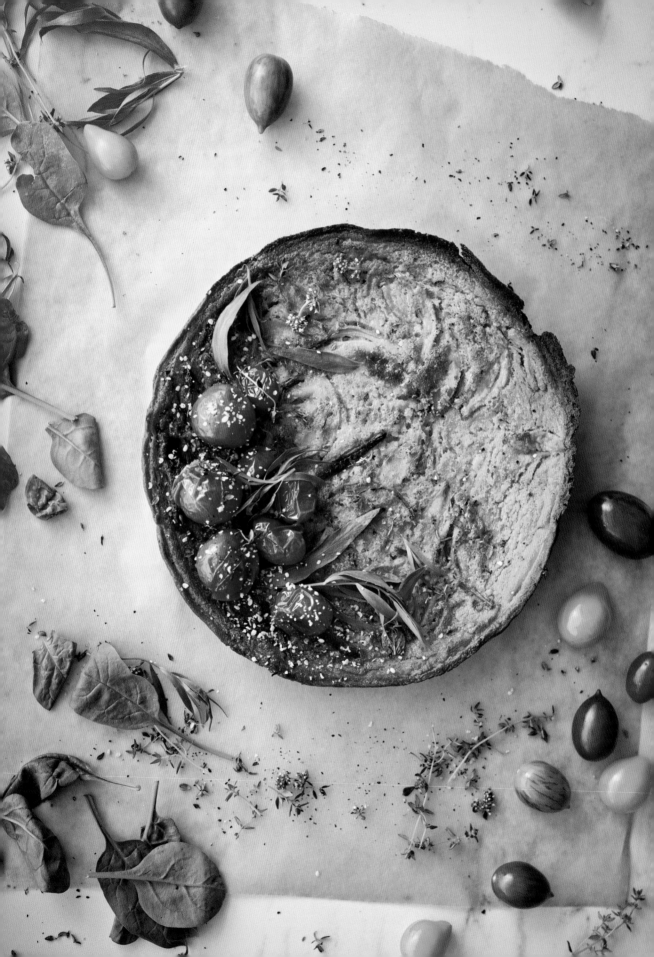

---

2 cups lukewarm water

1½ cups chickpea flour

1 shallot, thinly sliced

3 Tbsp avocado oil

1 tsp turmeric

2 tsp dried Italian seasoning

½ tsp sea salt

Pinch of pepper

1 Tbsp ghee

Extra Boosts:

Roasted cherry tomatoes

Hempy Pesto (page 243)

Chickpea flour, also known as garbanzo bean flour, can be found in health food stores and in most grocery stores, with the gluten-free flours.

Grain-Free Farinata Flatbread

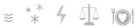

Farinata, also known as socca, is an Italian chickpea pancake that's a cross between a cracker and bread. It's thin, light, slightly dense, and oh so incredibly delicious. It can be eaten plain as is or used as a pizza crust or topped with avocado, roasted tomatoes, arugula, or our Hempy Pesto (page 243). This flatbread is wonderful if you have an upset stomach or if you're feeling nauseated. Because our farinata is made from chickpea flour, it's totally grain-free.

1. In a bowl, whisk together the warm water and chickpea flour until well combined. Once mixed, cover the bowl with a towel and allow the batter to rest for 30 minutes. It will thicken slightly.

2. When the batter has rested, heat the oven to 400°F and position a rack in the middle.

3. Whisk the shallots, avocado oil, Italian seasoning, turmeric, salt, and pepper into the batter.

4. Place a 10-inch cast iron pan, or a 10-inch oven-safe pan, over medium-high heat on the stove and add the ghee, swirling it around until the pan is well coated. Wear an oven mitt, as the handle may be hot.

5. Immediately pour the batter into the center of the pan. Swirl the batter around so that it coats the pan evenly.

6. Carefully transfer the pan to the oven and bake for 30 minutes, or until the edges of the farinata look crisp and the middle is slightly cracked. Allow it to cool for 5 minutes, then carefully use a spatula to remove the farinata from the pan and place it on a plate. You can eat it plain or top with roasted cherry tomatoes or Hempy Pesto.

7. Farinata is best when eaten hot, so eat it immediately, if you can. If you're eating it another day, store it in an airtight container in the fridge for up to 4 days and toast it before serving.

2 cups hazelnut flour

4 Tbsp virgin coconut oil, softened

½ cup dried currants

1 tsp dried rosemary

¼ tsp sea salt

Rosemary Currant Hazelnut Crackers

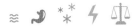

Crackers will be essential when you're going through treatment because they are helpful when your appetite is low. This is an easy recipe for crackers that are the perfect combo of sweet and salty flavors. Hazelnut flour is gluten-free and high in healthy fat and protein, making these crackers more nourishing than store-bought ones. The currants create a subtle sweetness balanced by the almost pine-like flavor of rosemary.

1. Preheat the oven to 325°F and line a baking sheet with parchment paper.
2. Blend all the ingredients in the food processor until they start to stick together as a dough. Remove the dough from the food processor and form it into a ball.
3. Put the dough between two sheets of parchment paper, and use a rolling pin (or a heavy glass bottle like a wine bottle or olive oil bottle) to roll out the dough as thin as you can. We like to aim for about ⅛ inch thick.
4. Use a knife to cut the dough into cracker shapes, like squares or rectangles, and carefully transfer these to the baking sheet.
5. Bake for 10–12 minutes, or until crisp on the edges and lightly browned on top. Watch these carefully, as they can easily burn.
6. Let the crackers cool down completely before storing in an airtight container. You can keep them for up to a week. Eat these with hummus, avocado, or coconut oil spread on top, or even on their own.

If you can't find hazelnut flour, you can easily make some at home. Simply blend 2 cups of raw hazelnuts in a food processor until they resemble flour. Just be careful to not over-process them into hazelnut butter. Then measure out 2 cups of flour.

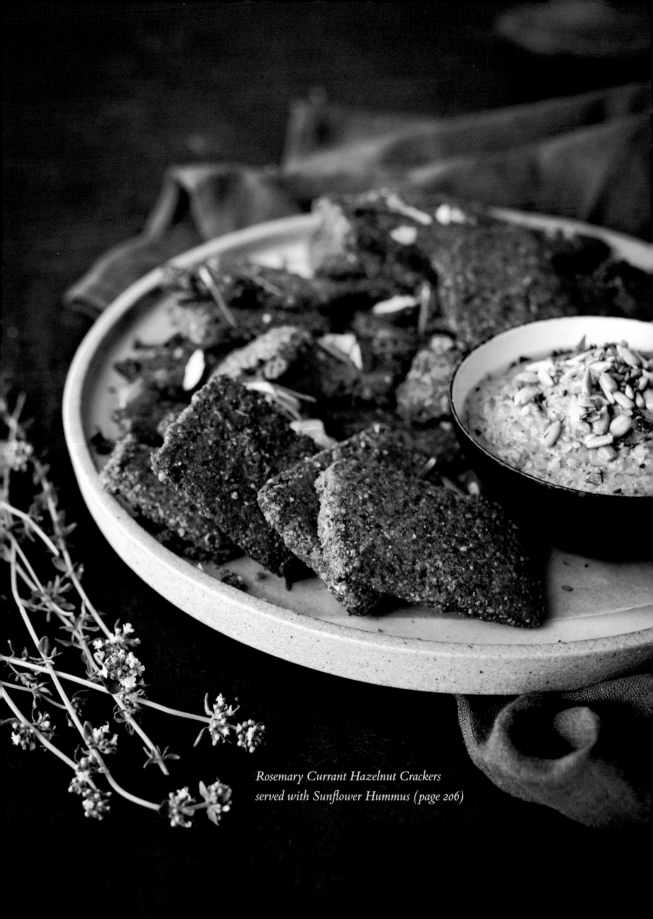

Rosemary Currant Hazelnut Crackers
served with Sunflower Hummus (page 206)

¼ cup raw sunflower seeds

4 Tbsp tahini

3–4 Tbsp cold water

3 Tbsp fresh lemon juice

2 Tbsp extra-virgin olive oil

2 Tbsp chopped fresh parsley

1 small garlic clove, minced

¼ tsp sea salt

Toppings:
Extra-virgin olive oil

Handful fresh parsley, chopped

Pinch of paprika

1 Tbsp sunflower seeds

NUTRITION NOTE Sunflower seeds contain selenium, a mineral that helps with DNA repair, so when you're going through treatment, it's an essential mineral for your diet.

Sunflower Hummus

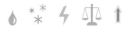

Many of our clients do not eat grains or legumes, but they still (understandably so!) want to enjoy foods they once loved, so we worked hard to develop a legume-free, Paleo-style hummus. Instead of chickpeas, we use sunflower seeds, which, when toasted, have a rich, nutty flavor and lend a smooth, creamy texture when blended up in the food processor. Eat this hummus with veggie sticks or with our Coconut Flour Biscuits (page 215).

1. Preheat the oven or toaster oven to 350°F and place the sunflower seeds on a small baking sheet lined with parchment paper. Toast in the oven for about 5 minutes, watching them carefully to make sure that they do not burn. Let the sunflower seeds cool for a few minutes.
2. Combine all the ingredients in the food processor and blend until smooth and creamy.
3. For the topping, drizzle with olive oil, and sprinkle fresh parsley, paprika, and sunflower seeds on top.
4. This hummus will keep in an airtight container in the fridge for 4 days.

½ cup raw almonds

½ cup raw Brazil nuts

½ cup raw pumpkin seeds

½ cup unsweetened coconut flakes, toasted if you prefer

⅓ cup cacao nibs

¼ cup dried golden berries or raisins

¼ cup dried goji berries

¼ cup dried mulberries

NUTRITION NOTE Almonds have a good amount of fat, protein, and fiber, and they supply energy and protect against free radicals. Pumpkin seeds will support your immune system. Brazil nuts contain selenium, a mineral necessary for detoxification. Cacao nibs naturally improve mood. Dried berries (golden, goji, and mulberry) are all antioxidant-rich.

Superfood Trail Mix

A special blend of crunchy raw chocolate and juicy dried fruit that bursts open like gummy candy is what makes this superfood trail mix so superbly super. You have almost certainly eaten a trail mix before, so you already know that it's an essential snack for giving you a quick energy boost, but good ol' raisins and peanuts (GORP) doesn't cut it anymore. Pair our revamped version with a bowl of yogurt, sprinkle it on top of a smoothie, or simply eat it right out of your hand.

1. Mix all the ingredients together in a large bowl.
2. Store in an airtight jar, in a cool dark spot, like a cupboard, for 1–2 months.

If you have trouble finding any of the berries called for in this recipe, they can easily be replaced with raisins and cranberries—just make sure they don't have any added sugar.

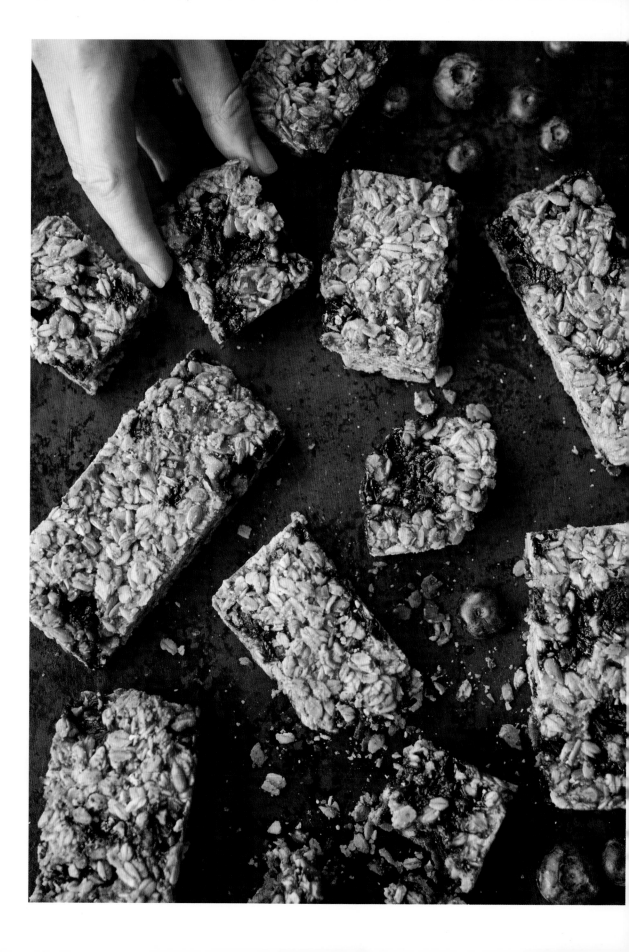

¼ cup virgin coconut oil

⅓ cup pure maple syrup

¼ cup almond butter

2 eggs

2 cups rolled oats

½ cup oat flour

¼ cup raw sunflower seeds

¼ cup raw walnut pieces

2 Tbsp lemon zest

2 Tbsp ground flaxseeds

1 cup fresh or frozen
    blueberries

If you can't find oat flour, feel free to use spelt or brown rice flour instead.

Zesty Blueberry Granola Bars

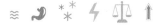

Granola bars are the ultimate on-the-go snack, which is essential when you need to fuel up during appointments and hospital visits. Making your own granola bars is fairly easy, inexpensive, and healthy, and we have the perfect recipe for you, one that is loaded with antioxidants, fiber, protein, and fat.

1. Preheat the oven to 350°F and line an 8- × 8-inch baking sheet with parchment paper.

2. Melt the coconut oil by placing it in a small pot on the stove top over medium-low heat until it liquefies. Remove it from the heat and stir in the maple syrup and almond butter.

3. In a large bowl, whisk together the eggs and add the coconut oil and maple syrup mixture. Make sure the coconut oil and maple syrup is only lukewarm so that it doesn't cook the eggs.

4. Combine the oats, oat flour, sunflower seeds, walnut pieces, lemon zest, and ground flaxseeds. Then fold this into the liquid ingredients, adding the blueberries. Mix well with a spoon. You may want to use your hands to help the sticky granola dough form.

5. Spread the mixture on the prepared pan, using your hands to spread and press it down evenly.

6. Bake in the oven for 30 minutes, or until the slab is firm and slightly brown on top.

7. Let cool for at least 30 minutes. Carefully lift the edges of the parchment paper to take the slab out of the pan. Then slice into bars.

8. You can store the granola bars in a container in the fridge for up to a week or freeze in an airtight container for up to 2 months.

---

1 banana, peeled and mashed

1 egg or 1 vegan egg (see recipe note)

¼ cup virgin coconut oil, melted

¼ cup pure maple syrup

1 cup oat flour or brown rice flour

¼ cup raw sunflower seeds

¼ cup raisins

¼ cup raw slivered almonds

¼ cup unsweetened shredded coconut

2 Tbsp vegan unsweetened protein powder

2 Tbsp hemp seeds

¾ tsp baking powder

½ tsp cinnamon

Pinch of sea salt

1 cup grated apple (Cortland, Empire, or Gala)

½ cup grated peeled carrots

3 Tbsp rolled oats

Apple Cinnamon Muffins

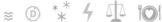

There are a lot of ingredients in these muffins, and they all have a purpose, adding sweetness, crunch, and a devious amount of good protein. These muffins will be slightly denser than you may be used to (I mean, they do use almost every ingredient in your kitchen!), but a baked item that's laced with maple syrup and almonds won't ever disappoint. A cinnamon- and apple-scented muffin that can be either a hearty snack or dessert is one you want in your repertoire. **TG**

1. Preheat the oven to 375°F and line a muffin tin with liners.
2. In a medium-sized bowl, combine the mashed banana, egg, coconut oil, and maple syrup.
3. In a large bowl, combine the flour, sunflower seeds, raisins, almonds, coconut, protein powder, hemp seeds, baking powder, cinnamon, and salt.
4. Pour the dry ingredients into the wet and mix well. Fold in the grated apple and carrots.
5. Scoop ½ cup of the batter into each cup, and top each one with a small sprinkle of oats. Then bake for 20–25 minutes, or until an inserted toothpick comes out clean and the top of each muffin is golden.
6. Store these in an airtight container in the fridge for up to a week or in the freezer for 2–3 months.

To make a vegan egg, mix 1 Tbsp of chia seeds or ground flaxseeds with 3 Tbsp of water and allow it to rest for 10 minutes, or until it becomes gelatinous.

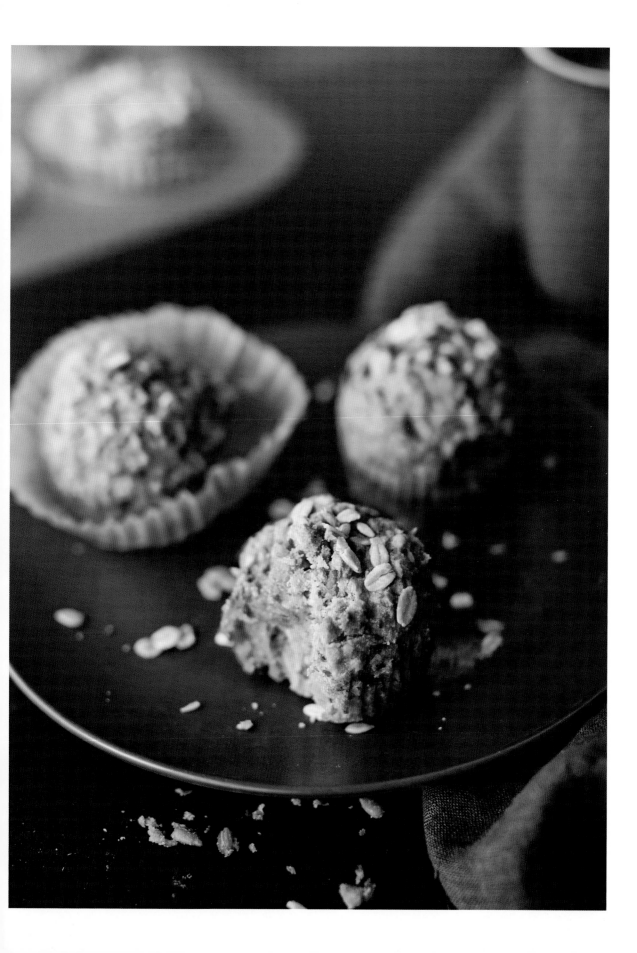

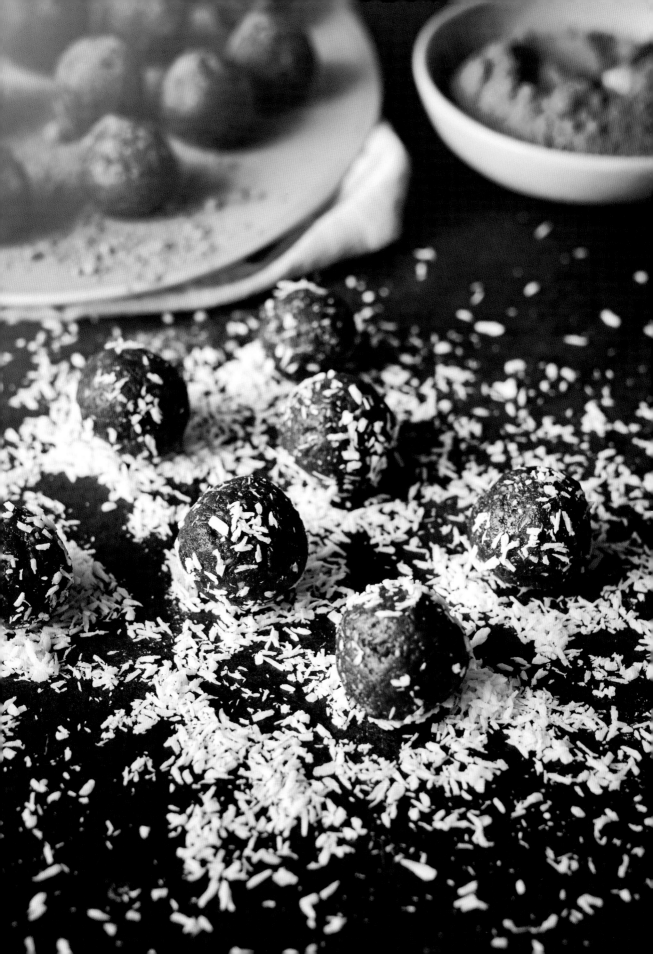

MAKES 24 BALLS

FREEZE: 2 MONTHS

PREP TIME: 20 MINUTES

1½ cups pitted dates

1 cup raw walnuts

½ cup raw sunflower seeds

½ cup raw cacao powder

½ tsp cinnamon

Pinch of sea salt

2 Tbsp virgin coconut oil, softened

1–2 Tbsp water (if needed)

1 cup unsweetened shredded coconut

Turmeric Power Truffles:

1 tsp turmeric

Pinch of pepper

Hemp Spirulina Power Truffles:

½ cup hemp seeds (this replaces the sunflower seeds at step 2)

½ tsp spirulina (this replaces the cinnamon at step 3)

Power Truffles

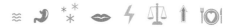

This is one of the most important recipes featured in this book—and not just because they taste like raw cookie dough brownies. Power truffles are portable bite-sized energy power-houses and easy to get down when you're having trouble eating. You always want to have a stash of these ready to go for a quick nutrition boost. And try the two variations we have on this recipe for something different.

1. Put the dates in warm water and allow them to soften for about 5 minutes. Drain and set aside.

2. Put the walnuts and sunflower seeds in a food processor and process until coarsely ground. If you are making Hemp Spirulina Power Truffles, use the hemp seeds instead of sunflower.

3. Add the cacao, cinnamon, and salt. If you are making Turmeric Power Truffles, add the turmeric and pepper. For Hemp Spirulina Power Truffles, replace the cinnamon with spirulina. Pulse a bit more, until the mixture is well combined.

4. Put the coconut oil and dates into the food processor and turn it on. A dough will begin to form. If the mixture is having a hard time blending and coming together, add the water, 1 tablespoon at a time, through the tube. Blend until the mixture is thick and sticky enough that it can be rolled into balls.

5. Take about 1 tablespoon of the dough and roll it into a ball. Continue until all the dough has been used.

6. Place the shredded coconut in a bowl and coat each ball in coconut. If you like, you can toast the coconut before rolling the balls in it.

7. Store in the fridge in an airtight container for up to 2 weeks or in the freezer for up to 2 months.

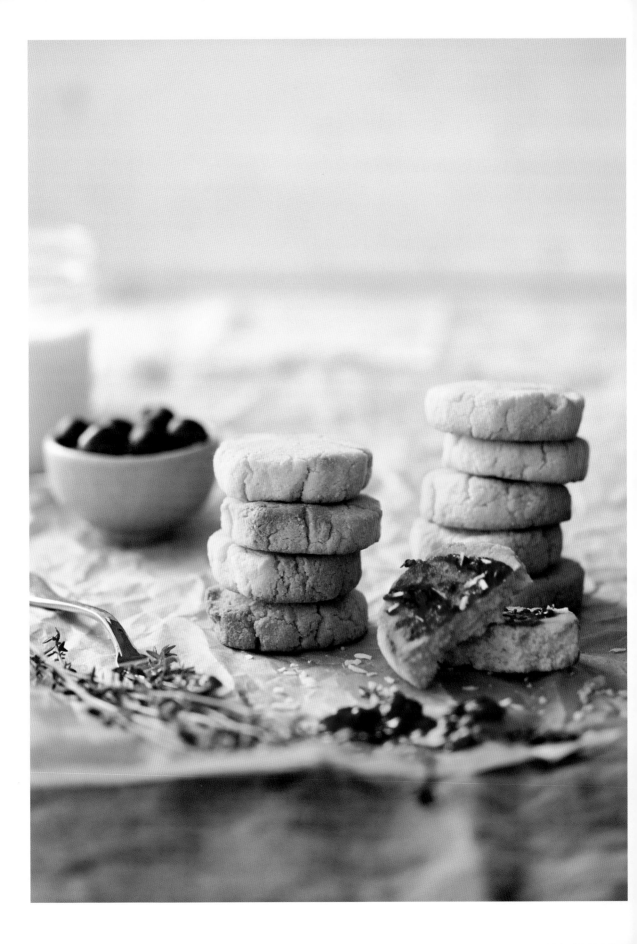

⅓ cup coconut flour

¼ cup virgin coconut oil, softened

1 egg

¼ tsp sea salt

NUTRITION NOTE Coconut flour is a great high-fiber, gluten-free, grain-free alternative to traditional flours, although it acts very differently than something like wheat flour. Coconut flour absorbs a significant amount of water, so you need only a small amount of it.

Coconut Flour Biscuits

Like everyone, sometimes we just crave bread, carbs, and baked goods. But if you're limiting your carb intake, you don't have a ton of choices when it comes to replacing these flour-based foods. We developed this biscuit recipe for a client who was following a carb-free diet during cancer treatment but still wanted something to eat that somewhat resembled biscuits. Without a doubt, this is one of the easiest recipes you'll find in our cookbook. Coconut flour has a naturally sweet flavor, which makes these biscuits savory with a hint of sweetness. These might seem plain, but they can be helpful if you feel nauseated and need a light snack to ease the stomach.

1. Preheat the oven to 350°F and line a baking sheet with parchment paper.
2. Put all the ingredients into a food processor and pulse until a dough forms. You can also mix the ingredients together in a bowl by hand.
3. Take 1 tablespoon of dough, roll it into a ball, and flatten. Continue to do this until all the dough has been used.
4. Place the biscuits on a baking sheet and bake for 12 minutes, or until they are slightly golden on top.
5. Let the biscuits cool completely before storing in an airtight container. You can keep them in the fridge for a few days. They taste best when warmed up.

Since they can be dry, these biscuits are best eaten with a drink. They are delicious served with our Sunflower Hummus (page 206) for a savory snack. Or spread them with fruit-juice-sweetened jam.

Masala Roasted Chickpeas

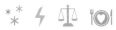

19 oz can chickpeas, or 1¼ cups cooked chickpeas

2 Tbsp extra-virgin olive oil

1 tsp garam masala

½ tsp cumin

½ tsp coriander

½ tsp granulated garlic powder

¼ tsp turmeric

¼ tsp sea salt

Perfectly crisp, salted, and boldly flavored, Masala Roasted Chickpeas are the most addictive snack in this entire cookbook. They're like chips or roasted nuts, and you'll eat them the very same way—by the handful. But guess what? Unlike chips—they're actually good for you! Roasting chickpeas together with these spices provides extra nutritional support by protecting your immune system. Step aside, potato chips, this new flavorful and healthy snack is taking over.

1. Preheat the oven to 350°F and line a baking sheet with parchment paper.
2. Drain and rinse a can of chickpeas. Pat them dry with a tea towel, making sure to remove as much liquid as possible, as they will roast better if they are dry.
3. In a large bowl, combine the oil with the spices and salt. Toss the chickpeas in the spices, making sure they are coated well.
4. Spread the seasoned chickpeas out on the baking sheet, then roast in the oven for 40 minutes, or until the chickpeas are crisp on the outside. After 20 minutes, gently shake the baking sheet to let the chickpeas roll around.
5. Remove from the oven and enjoy. You can put these on salads or on top of soups for added crunch, or eat them by the handful.
6. Store in a closed paper bag on the counter to keep them crisp for a week—but they may not last that long.

Once cooked, leftover chickpeas may get soft when stored. Pop them back in the oven at 350°F for 7 to 10 minutes to recrisp them.

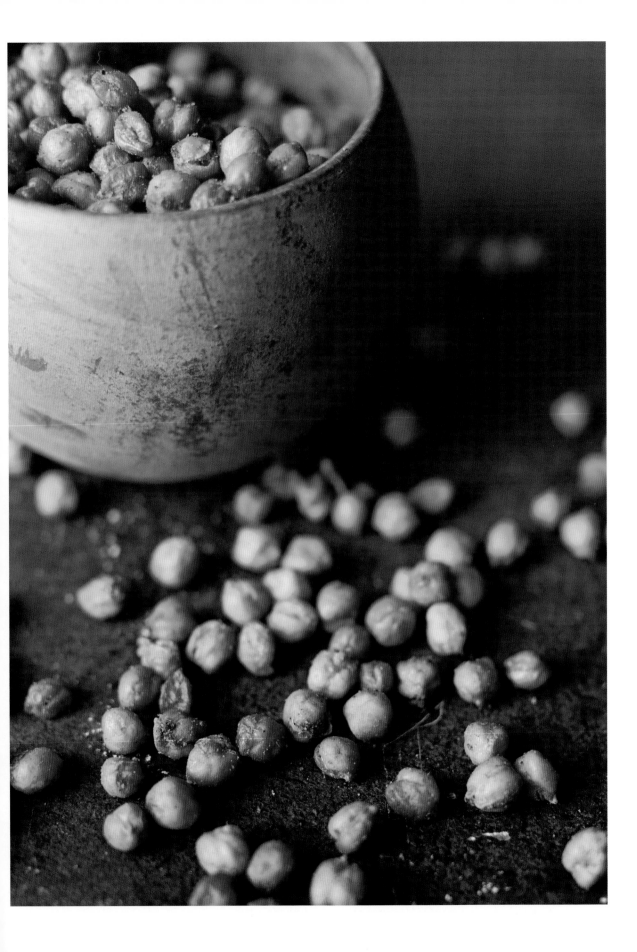

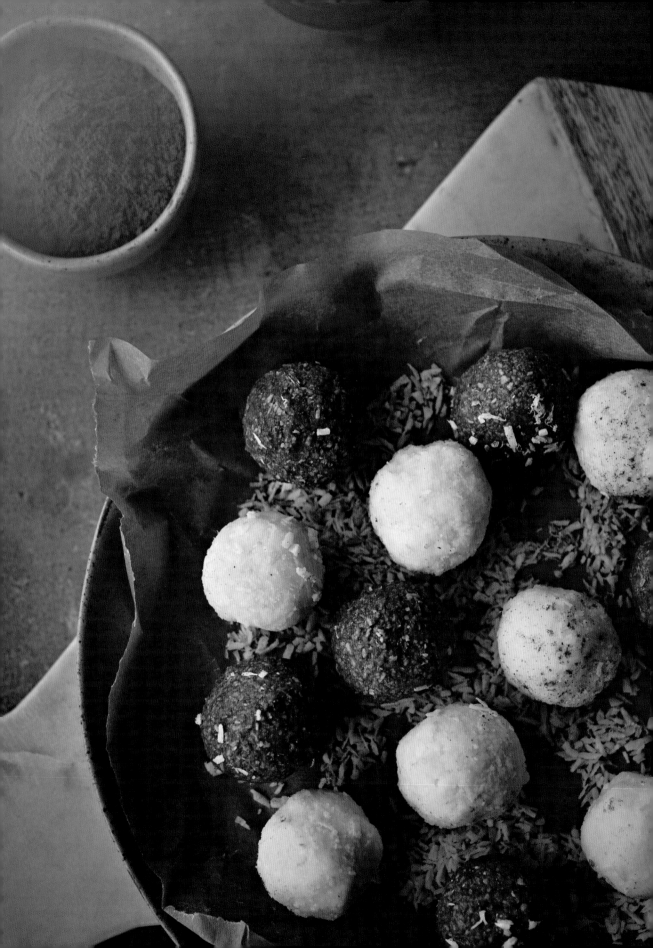

Base:

2 cups + ½ cup unsweetened finely shredded coconut, divided

3 Tbsp virgin coconut oil, softened

½ tsp pure vanilla extract

⅛ tsp stevia powder (add more or less, depending on preference)

Cacao Version:

2 Tbsp raw cacao powder

3 drops of mint extract or food-grade mint essential oil (optional)

Lemon Ginger Version:

2 tsp lemon zest (about 1 lemon)

½ tsp peeled and minced ginger root

Fat Bombs

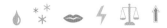

Fat bombs, eaten primarily in ketogenic diets, are high-fat, low-carb, low-protein snacks that allow you to eat a significant amount of fat in an easy and tasty way. These snacks are perfect if you have mouth sores, are having trouble chewing, or need something high in calories without eating a full meal. If you need to increase your fat intake, whether it's before surgery or during treatment, these will help with that.

We have two versions of this recipe. The base is the same, but you can choose which flavors to add. Cacao powder gives this snack a chocolaty flavor. Mint extract is optional, but if you love the classic chocolate-mint combo, we recommend it. Or try out lemon and ginger for a bright and uplifting flavor, with the perks of vitamin C and antinausea benefits of ginger.

1. To make the base, use a food processor to blend 2 cups of the shredded coconut and the coconut oil for about 2 minutes, until it becomes paste-like. You want the coconut pieces to blend all together. It's best if the coconut oil is slightly softened (but not melted), otherwise the mixture won't hold together as well. If you find it's too runny, you can place the coconut oil in the fridge for a few minutes to cool down.

2. Add the vanilla extract and stevia and pulse a few times to incorporate everything together. The mixture should be buttery and thick. To make the cacao version, add the cacao powder and mint extract. To make the lemon ginger version, add the lemon zest and ginger. Blend well to combine.

3. Remove the mixture from the food processor and scoop it into a large bowl. Stir in the ½ cup of reserved coconut.

4. Place the bowl in the fridge for 5 minutes to make the mixture stick together better.

continued

5. Use your hands to form the mixture into 10 balls. It will be sticky, so wet your hands slightly to prevent the balls from sticking to them.

6. Place in refrigerator for 30 minutes to firm up, then enjoy.

7. You can store these in the fridge for up to 1 month or in the freezer for 2–3 months. Let them warm up on the counter for 5–10 minutes before eating. If they are frozen, don't bite into them until they soften.

6 apples of choice, peeled
and cored (use a combo of
McIntosh, Cortland, Gala,
Fuji, and Golden Delicious)

¾ cup water

1 Tbsp fresh lemon juice

1 tsp cinnamon

¼ tsp ground cloves

⅛ tsp turmeric

Immune-Boosting Applesauce

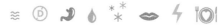

Imagine the fragrance of aromatic spices like cinnamon, cloves, and nutmeg swirling around your kitchen as applesauce simmers on the stove smelling like cider, Christmas, and winter all rolled into one. The scent alone will make you want to make this recipe. Applesauce is a must-have food for whenever you're not feeling well, as it soothes an upset stomach and a dry mouth. But here's what makes this recipe better than any store-bought version out there: the unique blend of spices specifically supports and protects your immune system while reducing inflammation. We like to use a variety of apples to hit on all those sweet, tart, and sour notes.

1. Cut the apples into large pieces and place them in a large pot, along with all the other ingredients and stir.
2. Bring the mixture to a boil, cover, and simmer on low heat for 20–30 minutes, or until the apples are soft.
3. After the time is up, stir the mixture with a wooden spoon. The apples will be so soft they will literally melt into each other and form a puree. If you like a smoother consistency, then puree it in a food processor once it cools. You may need to puree in two batches.
4. Store in an airtight container in the fridge for up to a week or in the freezer for up to 6 months. Eat it by the spoonful or on top of oatmeal, chia pudding, yogurt, or pancakes. You can also spread it on toast or add a few tablespoons to your favorite smoothie.

Make a big batch of this recipe and freeze it in small portions that can be easily reheated when you need an applesauce fix.

MAKES 6 LARGE MUFFINS

FREEZE: 2–3 MONTHS

PREP TIME: 10 MINUTES

COOK TIME: 30 MINUTES

---

1 small sweet potato, peeled

¼ cup extra-virgin olive oil

2 eggs

1½ cups chickpea flour

2 tsp baking powder

1 tsp dried rosemary

½ tsp sea salt

½ cup finely chopped spinach

½ cup finely chopped red pepper

½ cup finely chopped fresh basil

¼ cup raw pumpkin seeds

NUTRITION NOTE Chickpea flour is high in fiber and protein and contains iron, which is important for energy, and magnesium, essential for muscle relaxation. It's a good source of zinc, which has been linked with cancer prevention because of its important role in the proper function of DNA.

Chickpea Popkins

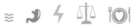

I was first introduced to savory muffins when I lived in New Zealand. Being accustomed to sweet muffins, I was initially skeptical, but ended up falling in love with their golden tops, tender veggies, and herbs. This new love inspired the creation of these popkins, a delicious gluten-free version of a savory muffin that pops with the fresh, bold flavor of basil. If you're having trouble eating veggies, this is the perfect snack, since the spinach and red pepper can be chopped very finely and, along with the pureed sweet potato, hidden within the batter. **SG**

1. Preheat the oven to 350°F, and line a muffin tin with liners. Coarsely chop the sweet potato into ½-inch cubes. Put them in a small pot, and add ½ cup of water so they're slightly covered but not drowning.
2. Cover the pot and put over medium heat for about 10 minutes, cooking until the sweet potato is soft. Once soft, mash the sweet potato with a fork or puree it in a food processor. Measure out ½ cup of mashed sweet potato.
3. In a bowl, whisk together the ½ cup of sweet potato, olive oil, and eggs.
4. In a separate bowl, combine the chickpea flour, baking powder, rosemary, and salt.
5. Pour the dry ingredients into the wet and gently mix to combine. Fold in the spinach, red pepper, and basil.
6. Scoop the batter among the muffin cups and sprinkle the pumpkin seeds on top.
7. Bake in the oven for 30 minutes, or until they are lightly browned on top and an inserted toothpick comes out clean.
8. These taste best when warmed up. We recommend enjoying them spread with some butter or ghee. You can store these in an airtight container in the fridge for 5 days or in the freezer for 2–3 months.

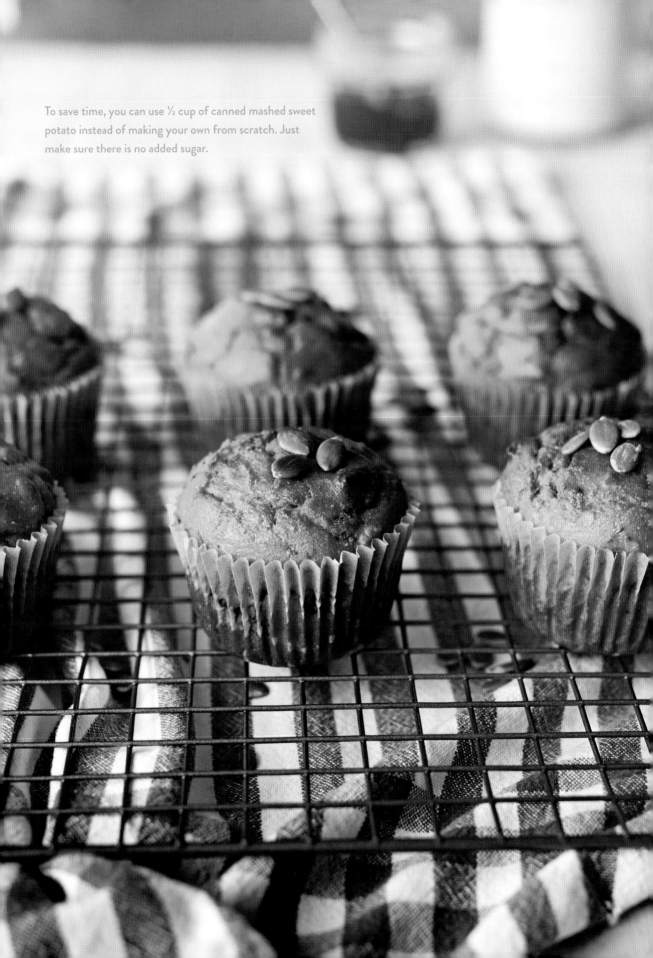

To save time, you can use ½ cup of canned mashed sweet potato instead of making your own from scratch. Just make sure there is no added sugar.

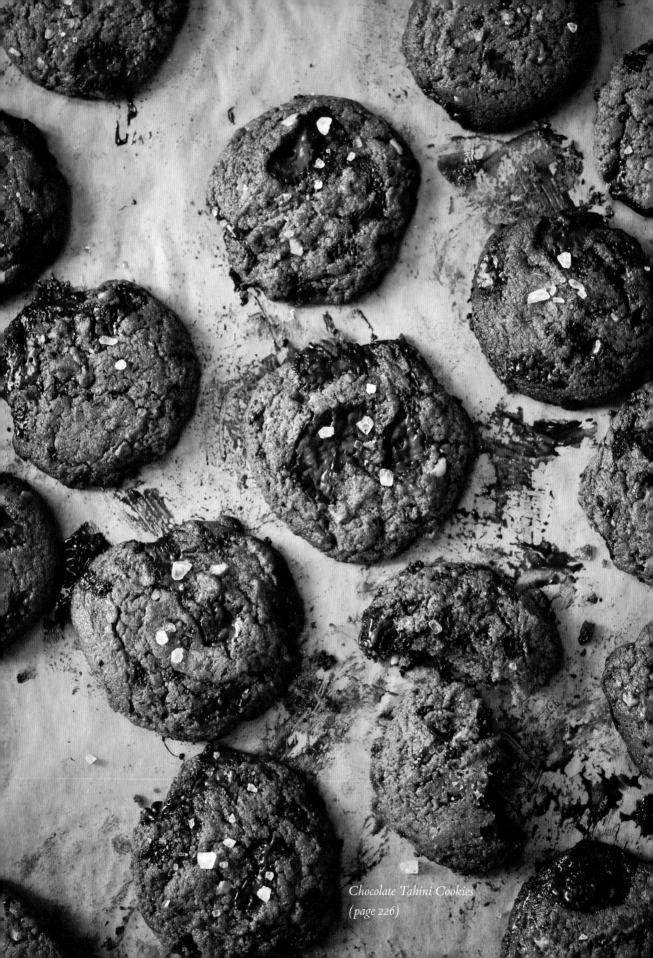

Chocolate Tahini Cookies
(page 226)

DESSERTS

You've made it to the sweetest chapter. Since we aren't the biggest fans of white flour or white sugar, these ingredients don't appear in any of our dessert recipes. We creatively use whole, natural ingredients like dates, raw cacao, berries, and almonds to make indulgent and decadent desserts that will satisfy any and all sweet cravings, *and* support your body during and after treatment.

———————

1 large egg

½ cup tahini

½ cup blanched almond flour

½ cup coconut sugar

½ tsp baking powder

One 3.5 oz 70% (or higher) dark chocolate bar, coarsely chopped

¼ tsp coarse sea salt

NUTRITION NOTE Almond flour is low glycemic, yet has a naturally sweet flavor. It is higher in protein and fat than grain-based flours, which will help keep blood sugar stable, especially while eating cookies.

Chocolate Tahini Cookies

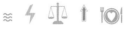

You simply cannot have a dessert chapter without including a recipe for chocolate chip cookies. This recipe has been tried and tested more times than we can remember and is a longtime favorite of many clients, who make them every week as a staple snack to keep on hand. Similar to our other desserts, these cookies are gluten-free because we use tahini and almond flour as the base rather than traditional white flour, making sure you get all the nutrients you need before, during, and after treatment.

1. Preheat the oven to 350°F and line a baking sheet with parchment paper.
2. In a medium-sized bowl, mix together the egg, tahini, almond flour, coconut sugar, and baking powder. It will make a thick, sticky mixture.
3. Fold in the chopped chocolate.
4. Scoop about 1 tablespoon of batter and place it on the baking sheet. Continue to do this, spacing each cookie about 2½ inches apart, until you have used all of the dough. If you prefer a larger cookie, scoop 2 tablespoons per cookie. Sprinkle cookies with the coarse salt.
5. Bake in the oven for 8–9 minutes, watching carefully because they can burn easily. They should be just lightly browned on top.
6. Let cool for 10 minutes on the baking sheet. Then transfer to a plate or container for storage.
7. These can be stored in a cool place in the pantry for 2 days or in the fridge for 1 week. You can freeze these for 3–4 months.

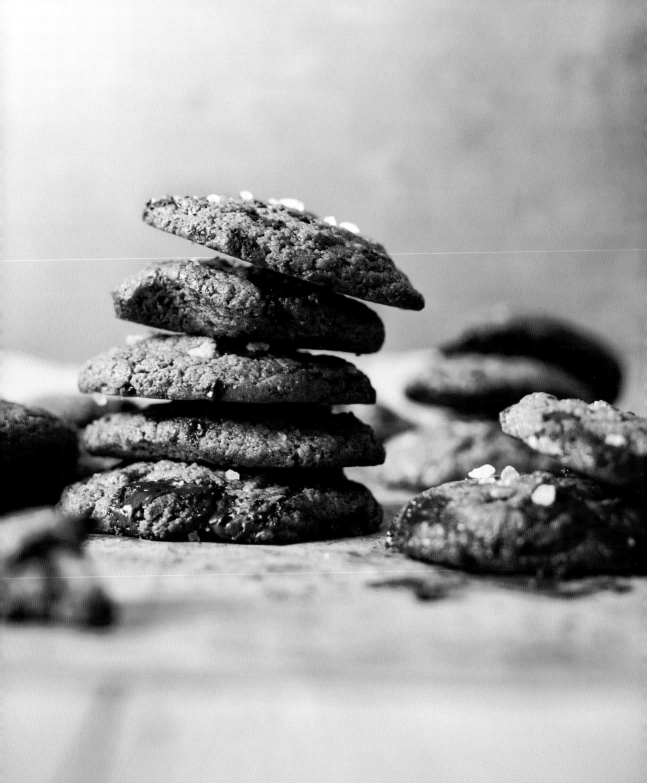

---

1 cup puffed quinoa

1 cup walnuts, coarsely chopped

1 cup + 2 Tbsp unsweetened shredded coconut, divided

½ cup raw pumpkin seeds

½ cup hemp seeds

1 cup nut or seed butter of choice

⅓ cup honey

1 Tbsp + 2 tsp virgin coconut oil, divided

2 cups 70% (or higher) dark chocolate chips

¼ tsp coarse sea salt

Sea Salt Quinoa Chocolate Bars

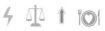

These bars might just change your life. Unlike traditional chocolate bars that are made with refined sugar, glucose syrup, artificial flavoring, and vegetable oils, these ones are made with "superfood" ingredients and are sweetened naturally. Every bite brings crunch, together with sweet, salty, and decadent flavor. These bars are hearty, so a little goes a long way.

1. Combine the puffed quinoa, walnuts, 1 cup of the coconut flakes, pumpkin seeds, and hemp seeds in a bowl.
2. Place a large pot on the stove over medium heat and add the nut butter, honey, and 1 tablespoon of the coconut oil, stirring constantly with a silicone spatula. When it turns slightly bubbly and smooth, add the puffed quinoa mixture and stir well to combine.
3. Line a 9- × 9-inch baking dish with parchment paper and scoop the mixture in. Allow it to cool slightly and then press it down to spread and flatten. Place it in the fridge for 15 minutes.
4. Melt the chocolate chips with the 2 teaspoons of coconut oil in a double boiler, stirring with a silicone spatula until smooth. Carefully pour the melted chocolate over the quinoa mixture. Spread it out using the spatula.
5. Sprinkle the top with the remaining shredded coconut and the salt. Place in the fridge for 1 hour, until firm.
6. Lift the slab out of the pan and, using a sharp knife, cut into squares. The bars may crumble slightly as you cut.
7. Store in an airtight container in the fridge for a week or freezer for up to 1 month.

Puffed quinoa is exactly what it sounds like: quinoa that's been puffed, similar to puffed rice. You can find it at health food stores, online, or in some grocery stores. It provides a soft crunch while also offering fiber, protein, and B vitamins.

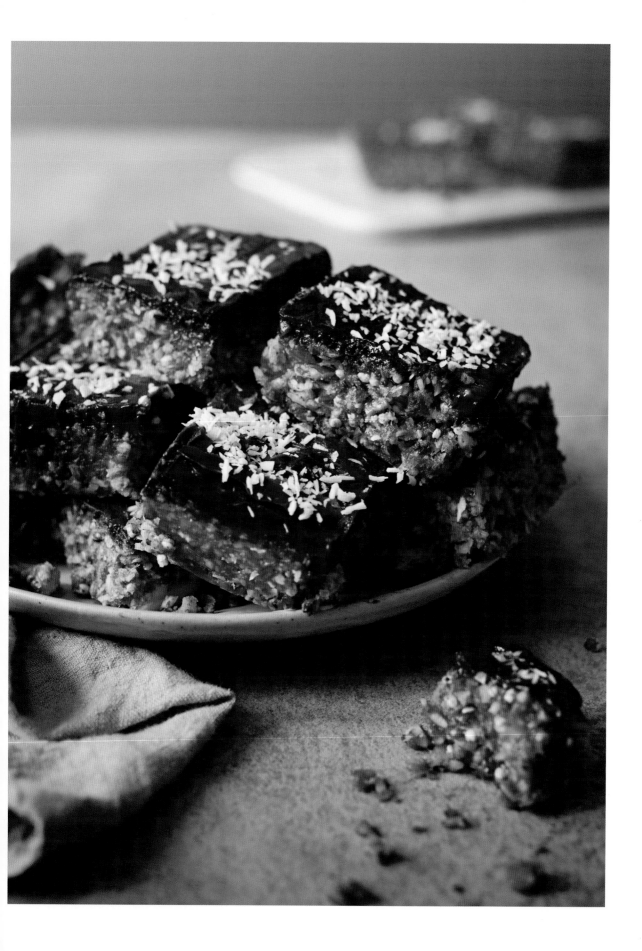

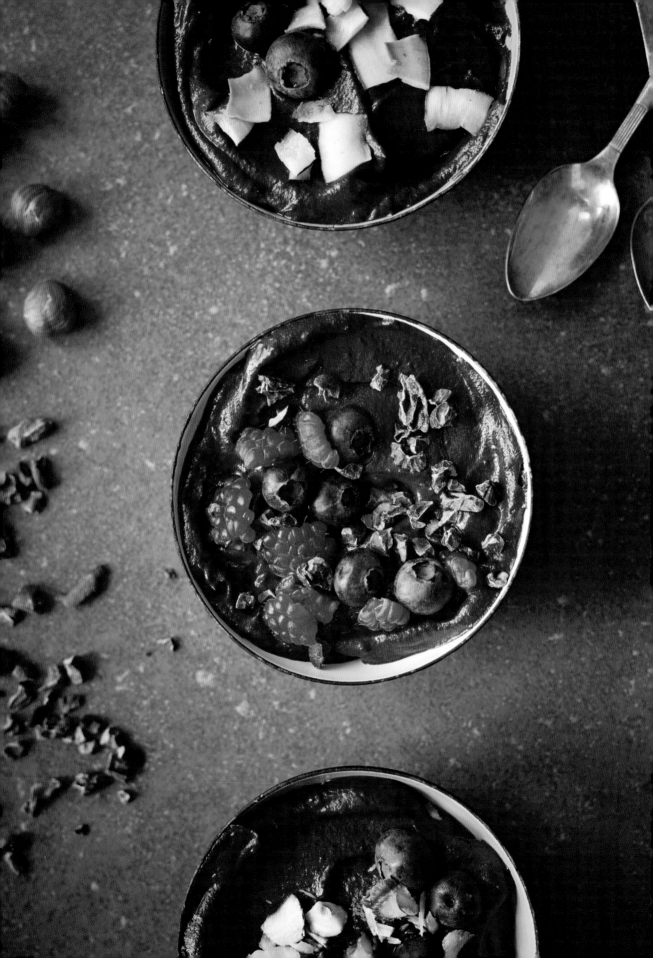

MAKES 2 SERVINGS

PREP TIME: 10 MINUTES

¼ cup packed pitted dates

2 ripe avocados

¼ cup unsweetened dairy-free milk

¼ cup raw cacao powder

½ tsp pure vanilla extract

Pinch of sea salt

Toppings:

Berries or fruit of your choice

Unsweetened coconut flakes

80% dark chocolate chips

Chopped raw pecans, walnuts, or almonds

Cacao nibs

Hemp seeds

Goji berries

Mint leaves

Cinnamon

Raw cacao powder for dusting

Avocado Chocolate Mousse

Avocados are not just for guacamole; they are versatile chameleons. Spread them on toast, blend them into smoothies, and even use them in desserts, like our Avocado Chocolate Mousse. This recipe was our first introduction to using avocados in desserts, and it's been a winner ever since. Here, avocado is the secret ingredient—this mousse is so chocolaty, soft, and silky, you will never know that it's not made from real cream.

1. Soak the dates in a bowl of warm water for 5 minutes. Once they've softened, drain the water.
2. Blend the dates, avocados, dairy-free milk, cacao powder, vanilla extract, and salt in a food processor until the mixture becomes creamy and smooth. If you have trouble getting the mixture to blend, gradually add a bit more milk, one spoonful at a time.
3. Divide between two bowls, garnish with whichever toppings you like, and enjoy!
4. Store in the fridge for up to 2 days in an airtight container.

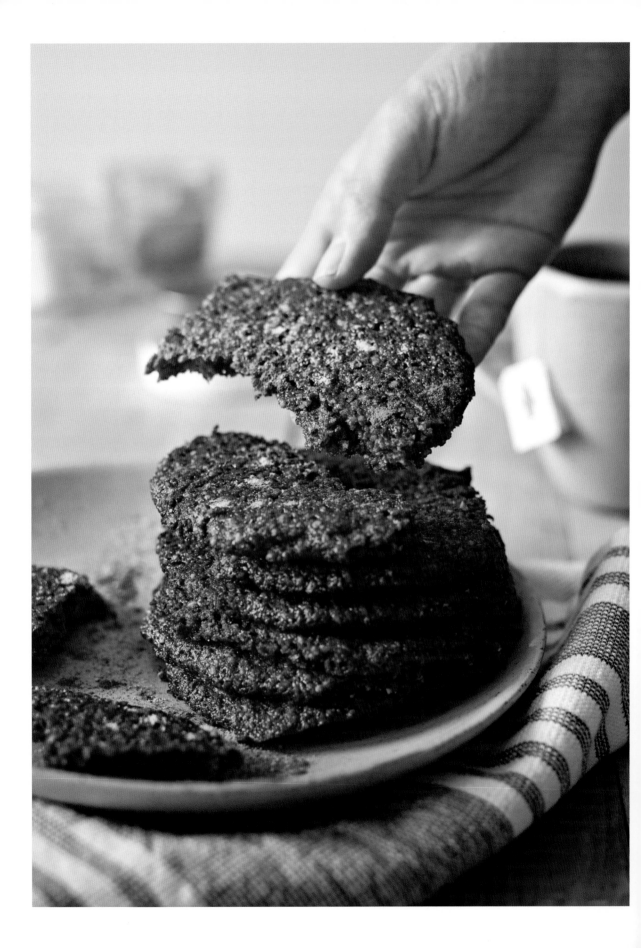

MAKES 12 COOKIES

FREEZE: 3–4 MONTHS

PREP TIME: 15 MINUTES

COOK TIME: 13 MINUTES

¼ cup virgin coconut oil

1½ cups hazelnut flour

¼ cup coconut sugar

1 tsp cinnamon

½ tsp baking soda

Small pinch of sea salt

1 egg

3 Tbsp dark unsulfured blackstrap molasses

2 tsp minced or finely grated peeled ginger root

NUTRITION NOTE Ginger and cinnamon are both appetite stimulants. Ginger is known to ease an upset stomach.

Gingersnap Cookies

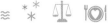

When my mom was pregnant with me, instead of eating red meat, she'd eat a tablespoon of blackstrap molasses every day to keep her iron levels up. Because of that, I've always loved mineral-rich molasses, and I try to find ways to integrate it into recipes. These cookies are full of delicious spices that immediately make us feel warm and cozy. Plus, they have the perfect cookie combination of crisp on the outside and soft and chewy on the inside. **SG**

1. Preheat the oven to 350°F and line a baking sheet with parchment paper.
2. Warm the coconut oil in a pot over low heat until just melted. Remove the pot from the heat immediately and let cool slightly.
3. In a bowl, combine the hazelnut flour, coconut sugar, cinnamon, baking soda, and salt.
4. In a large bowl, place the egg, molasses, ginger root, and melted coconut oil and whisk them together.
5. Pour the dry ingredients into the wet and mix with a spoon until a dough forms.
6. Scoop out 1 tablespoon of dough, place on the baking sheet, and flatten. Continue until all the dough has been used, keeping the cookies about 2 inches apart.
7. Bake the cookies for 13 minutes. The cookies will spread out a bit and be crisp on the edges.
8. Let cool for 10 minutes on the baking sheet before eating.
9. These can be stored in a cool place in the pantry for 2 days or in the fridge for 1 week. You can freeze these for 3–4 months.

If you don't have hazelnut flour, you can use almond flour instead.

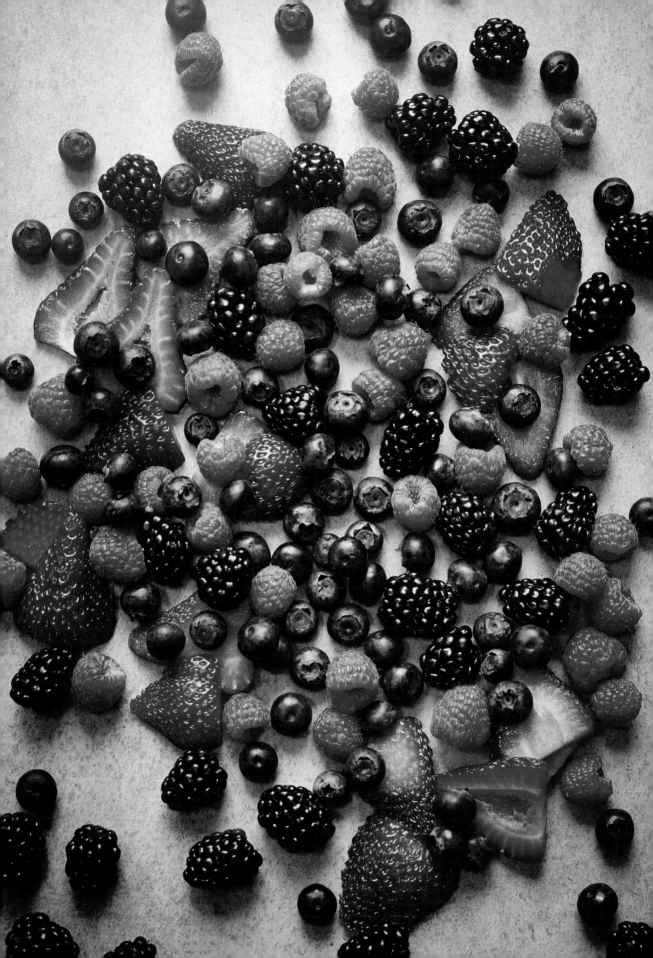

MAKES 6–8 SERVINGS

FREEZE: 3–4 MONTHS

PREP TIME: 15–20 MINUTES

COOK TIME: 30 MINUTES

Filling:

2 Granny Smith apples, sliced into thin wedges

2 cups fresh or frozen berries of your choice

½ lemon, juiced

Topping:

2 cups unsweetened coconut flakes

1 cup raw pecans, chopped

½ tsp cinnamon

Pinch of sea salt

3 Tbsp pure maple syrup

3 Tbsp virgin coconut oil, softened

2 Tbsp tahini

Baked Apple Berry Crumble

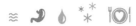

Although I always love chocolate-based desserts, I would eat this crumble after any meal, and I'd even eat it for breakfast, since it's not too sweet. There's something about warm baked fruit that's so delicious—the fruit becomes sweeter and melts in your mouth, and when it's paired with a crispy topping, it makes for a divine combination of textures. The grain-free topping in this recipe uses tahini and shredded coconut as its base, rather than traditional oats, which makes for a delicious spin on a classic. Plus, our version is low-glycemic and provides healthy fats that you'll need to keep calorie intake up during your cancer therapy. **SG**

1. Preheat the oven to 350°F and line a 9-inch pie dish or 8- × 8-inch baking dish with parchment paper.

2. To make the filling, in a large bowl, toss the apples and berries together with the lemon juice.

3. To make the topping, in another bowl, add the coconut flakes, pecans, cinnamon, and salt, and mix them together. Then add the maple syrup, softened coconut oil, and tahini, and stir. Use your hands to mix the ingredients to form a crumbly mixture.

4. Pour the filling into the prepared dish and spread it out evenly. Sprinkle the topping over the filling.

5. Bake in the oven for 30 minutes, or until the fruit is bubbling and soft and the topping is lightly browned. If the topping looks as if it is going to burn, cover it with tinfoil.

6. Baked Apple Berry Crumble is delicious served with a scoop of coconut yogurt or coconut milk whipped cream for a dairy-free treat. Store this in the fridge for up to 4 days or in the freezer for 3–4 months.

For a more traditional grain-based version of crumble, use 2 cups of rolled oats instead of unsweetened coconut flakes.

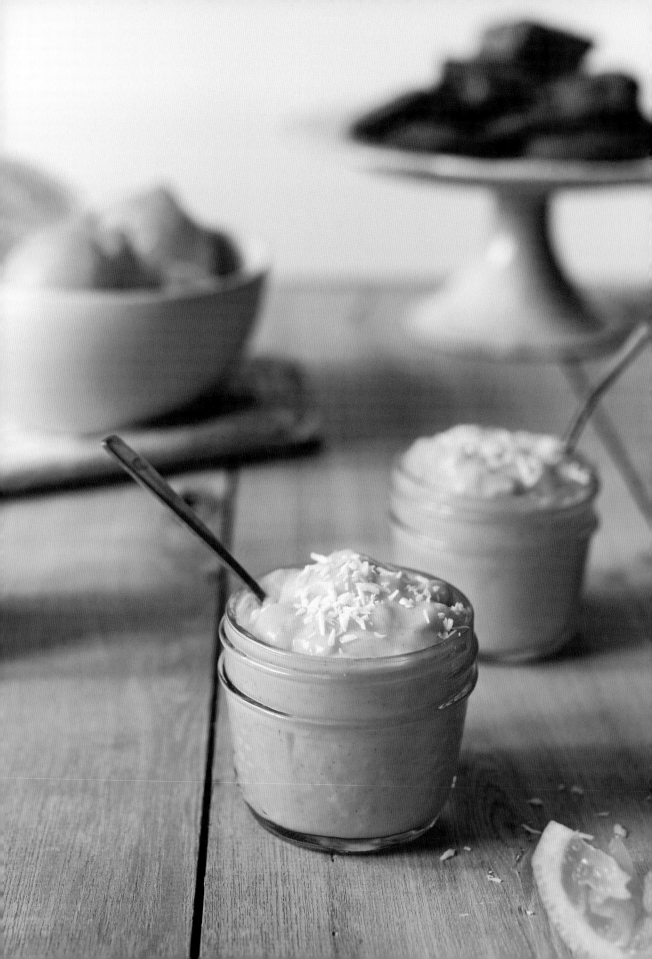

---

14 oz can full-fat coconut milk

¼ cup fresh lemon juice

2 Tbsp pure maple syrup

1½ Tbsp lemon zest

½ tsp turmeric

¼ cup arrowroot powder

Extra Boosts:
Shredded coconut

Berries

NUTRITION NOTE Lemons
help stimulate saliva production
and appetite, and they are a
great source of vitamin C.

Lemon Custard

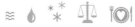

Creamy coconut milk can taste quite decadent and rich, but luckily it won't leave you feeling bloated or congested like dairy might. Zesty lemon makes a refreshing dessert here that's creamy, tangy, and sweet, and can help if you have altered taste buds. Turmeric powder makes this dish anti-inflammatory and creates a beautiful, bright-yellow color that's unlike any other dessert!

1. In a small pot, add the coconut milk, lemon juice, maple syrup, lemon zest, and turmeric and mix. Add the arrowroot powder and whisk well, making sure that the mixture is smooth and that there are no clumps.

2. Set the pot over medium heat, stirring occasionally to prevent the arrowroot from clumping. Once the mixture begins to bubble, reduce the heat to low and simmer for 5 minutes, stirring often to prevent the mixture from burning on the bottom of the pot. The mixture will start to thicken after 5 minutes of being heated. It will have a custard-like consistency at this point but will not be set.

3. Pour the mixture into a bowl, or alternatively, you can portion the mixture out into small mason jars. Let the mixture cool in the fridge for 1 hour. As it cools, the custard will set.

4. You can store this in the fridge for 4 days in an airtight container. We find this recipe most refreshing when it's cold, but you can also let it warm up on the counter to room temperature before eating. You can top the custard with some shredded coconut or berries before serving.

You can make this recipe completely sugar-free by using stevia instead of maple syrup. Add around 6 drops of stevia, to your taste preference.

¼ cup virgin coconut oil

19 oz can chickpeas, drained and rinsed or 2¼ cups cooked chickpeas

3 eggs

½ cup coconut sugar

1 tsp baking powder

Pinch of sea salt

¾ cup 70% (or higher) dark chocolate chips or one 3.5 oz 70% (or higher) dark chocolate bar, coarsely chopped

Chickpea Chocolate Chip Blondies

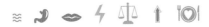

Blondies made out of chickpeas may sound strange, but trust us, they're divine. The chickpeas give these bars a fudgy consistency and also offer more protein than your average dessert, so it's an excellent snack and energy booster. Chocolate chunks crack through the smooth top golden layer and billow out, so every bite is chocolate-filled. Pair this treat with a big mug of our Olympic Gold Milk (page 90), for when you need something a little special.

1. Preheat the oven to 350°F, and line an 8- × 8-inch baking dish with parchment paper, draping extra over the edges to act as handles.
2. Place the coconut oil in a pot over low heat until just melted. Remove from the heat and let it cool slightly.
3. Put all the ingredients except for the chocolate chips in a food processor or a high-speed blender and blend until the mixture has a smooth, creamy consistency, then pour into a separate bowl.
4. Using a spatula or wooden spoon, fold in the chocolate chips.
5. Pour the blondie batter into the baking dish. Smooth the top with a spatula and shake the pan until the batter is evenly spread out.
6. Bake for 30 minutes, or until the center is solid to the touch and the top is golden.
7. Gently lift the slab out by pulling up the parchment paper and setting it on the counter. Once cooled, slice into 16 squares.
8. These blondies can be stored in an airtight container in the fridge for 4 days or in the freezer for up to 1 month.

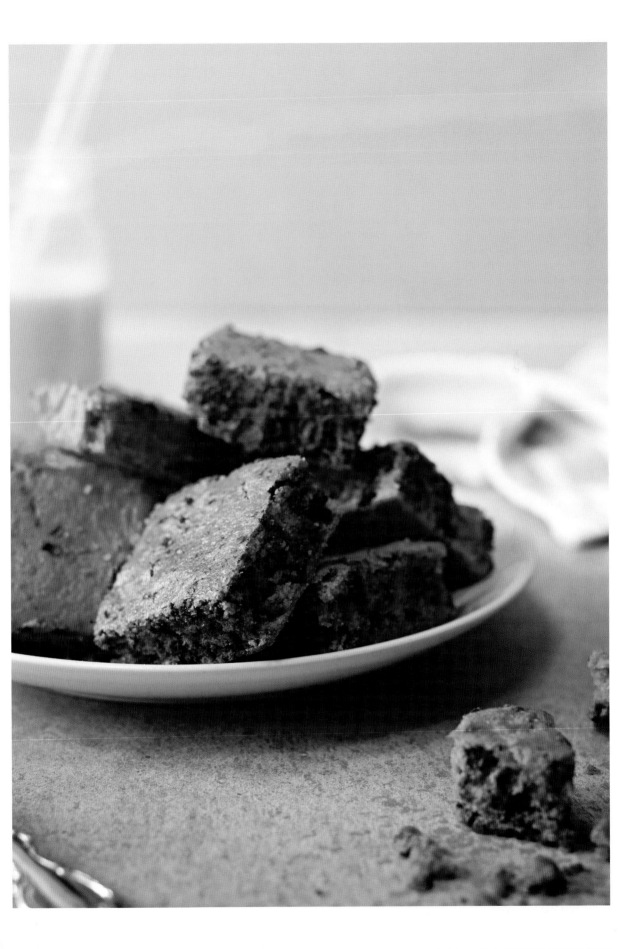

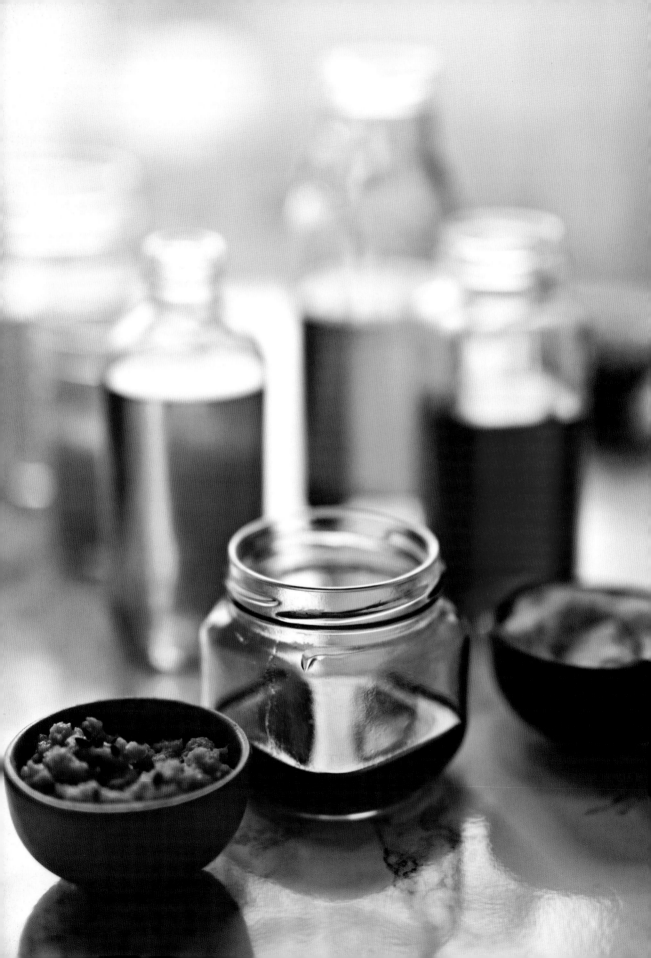

SAUCES, MARINADES, AND DRESSINGS

Sauces, marinades, and dressings help to amplify almost any dish. It's easy to buy condiments from the store, but they're usually loaded with refined sugars, vegetable oils, and preservatives. Our recipes are nutritious, quick, easy, tasty, and add additional fat and moisture. This is especially helpful if you're low on energy and you need extra calories for weight gain, and if you're suffering from the common cancer treatment side effects of compromised taste buds, sore mouth, and reduced saliva production.

¼ cup tahini

2 Tbsp tamari, or coconut
aminos (if you don't eat soy)

4 tsp pure maple syrup

2 tsp grated or minced peeled
ginger root

Water for thinning, if needed

Tahini Tamari Swirl

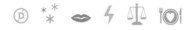

Nutty tahini swirled with spicy ginger, salty tamari, and maple come together to make an Asian-inspired sauce that will enhance any dish you slather it on. Eat it with our Rainbow Wraps (page 161); drop dollops on top of chicken, fish, beans, cooked veggies, or raw salads; or, if you feel so inclined, just dig in with a spoon.

1. Combine all the ingredients together in a bowl and mix well until a creamy, caramel-colored sauce forms.
2. This is a thicker sauce, almost resembling the consistency of a marinade, so if you like a thinner sauce, add a few spoonfuls of water.
3. Keep it in an airtight container in the fridge for up to a week.

Tamari is the traditionally brewed version of soy sauce. Most soy sauces found at grocery stores use GMO soybeans and caramel coloring and are produced quickly, so they don't undergo the proper fermentation period.

Coconut aminos, made from coconuts, are a completely soy-free alternative to soy sauce. Both tamari and coconut aminos are fermented for a longer time and can be made without wheat or gluten.

---

1 cup packed fresh basil leaves

1 garlic clove, coarsely chopped

¼ cup hemp seeds

¼ cup extra-virgin olive oil

¼ cup hemp oil

1 Tbsp fresh lemon juice

¼ tsp sea salt

Pinch of pepper

NUTRITION NOTE Omega-3-rich hemp oil not only helps reduce inflammation but also has been linked with slowing cancer cell replication. It's important to remember that this pesto cannot be heated because that would damage the hemp oil. Hemp oil, like all omega-3-rich oils, loses its nutritional health benefits when heated. So just add this pesto to dishes after cooking.

Hempy Pesto

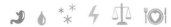

One of my favorite things to do in summer is hike over to the local farmers' market near our home to buy freshly picked basil. I love coming home, proudly putting the basil in a vase, and letting the fresh scent fill the kitchen for a couple of days before whipping up a batch of this pesto. Although classic pesto is made with pine nuts, we've switched it up and use hemp seeds instead to amp up the omega-3 fat content. This pesto is used in our Pesto Sweet Potato Chicken Salad (page 136). **SG**

1. Pluck the basil leaves off the stems and rinse the leaves under cold water to remove any soil. Dry the leaves as much as possible. You can use a salad spinner or pat the leaves dry with a tea towel.
2. Add all the ingredients to the food processor and pulse until the basil leaves, garlic, and hemp seeds are finely chopped.
3. Store the pesto in an airtight container in the fridge for up to a week or freeze for up to 1 year.

If you aren't going to use up the pesto when it's fresh, you can freeze it. Our favorite way to freeze pesto is in an ice-cube tray. Once frozen, you can pop the pesto cubes out when you need them. They'll keep in the freezer for up to a year.

If you don't have hemp oil you can replace it with extra-virgin olive oil.

---

1 cup cucumber

1 garlic clove, minced

1 cup plain, unsweetened
coconut yogurt

¼ cup fresh dill, finely chopped

1 Tbsp lemon juice

¼ tsp sea salt

Coconut Tzatziki

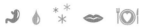

We came up with this spin on tzatziki using dairy-free coconut yogurt instead of regular yogurt to avoid the inflammatory properties of dairy. The bite of garlic, fresh dill, and tart lemon juice blend together to create a refreshing sauce that barely tastes like coconut. And our clients who can't eat dairy can still enjoy tzatziki. We like to pair this with our Dill Salmon Burgers (page 149).

1. Grate the cucumber with a hand grater or in a food processor using the grater attachment.
2. In a medium-sized bowl, combine the grated cucumber with all the other ingredients.
3. Keep chilled in the refrigerator until ready to use or serve. This tzatziki will keep in an airtight container in the fridge for up to 4 days.

Make sure to buy yogurt that is made of coconut milk (not dairy yogurt with a coconut flavor). Alternatively, you can use another type of dairy-free yogurt, such as almond milk yogurt. Just make sure you get an unsweetened, plain variety.

————————

2 Tbsp white miso

2 Tbsp toasted sesame oil

2 Tbsp water

4 tsp tahini

4 tsp extra-virgin olive oil

2 tsp maple syrup

NUTRITION NOTE Miso has
been shown to inhibit the growth
of most hormone-dependent
cancers (like breast, ovarian, and
prostate), and toasted sesame oil
provides healthy fat.

Miso Sesame Sauce

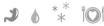

Miso is one of our favorite condiments to use in our recipes
because it lends a creamy texture to sauces and marinades, and it's
naturally very salty but also subtly sweet. Throwing sesame oil
into the mix brings out a toasted flavor. This sauce is delicious
drizzled over veggies, rice, or soba noodles. You can also use it
in our Rainbow Wraps (page 161).

1. Whisk together all the ingredients or blend them up in
   a food processor.
2. If the sauce is too thick, gradually add a few spoonfuls
   of water to thin it out.
3. Store it in an airtight container in the fridge for up to
   a week.

If you don't eat soy, look for miso that's made out of chickpeas, instead
of soybeans, at your local health food store or online.

----

3 Tbsp full-fat coconut milk

¼ cup almond butter

1 Tbsp fresh lime juice

2 tsp tamari, or coconut aminos
(if you don't eat soy)

2 tsp maple syrup

Pinch of cayenne (optional)

Almond Coconut Lime Sauce

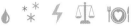

While venturing through Thailand I took part in a Thai cooking class in Chiang Mai. I was put on satay duty, which meant vigorously crushing spices and peanuts with a mortar and pestle. Luckily, this step is not required in our recipe here. This sauce is inspired by that tasty experience, with a few modifications. We've swapped out peanuts and replaced them with almond butter. The sauce is naturally sweet, with a good amount of zip from the tamari and zesty lime juice. Drizzle it over our Simple Sushi Bowl (page 164), or use it as a dipping sauce for chicken or veggies. **TG**

1. If you are opening a fresh can of coconut milk, incorporate the coconut cream that sits on top by mixing it well within the can so a thick liquid forms. You can use the leftover milk in many of our smoothie recipes.
2. Place all of the ingredients together in the food processor or blender and blitz until the mixture has a creamy consistency.
3. Store in an airtight container; it keeps in the fridge for up to 5 days.

————————

3 Tbsp water

2 Tbsp tahini or almond butter

2 Tbsp extra-virgin olive oil

2 Tbsp fresh lemon juice

2 tsp maple syrup

1 tsp turmeric

½ tsp minced peeled ginger
  root

¼ tsp minced garlic

¼ tsp sea salt

Pinch of pepper

Golden Turmeric Sauce

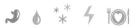

For the last couple of years, we've participated in a big foodie catering event that raises money for breast cancer research. The dish we were making at last year's event needed a sauce, and through a complete kitchen mishap we accidentally created Golden Turmeric Sauce. We fell in love. The color is a bright fiery yellow, and the taste is a bit spicy from the ginger but rounded out with sweetness from the maple syrup. Use this sauce on top of quinoa or brown rice, with cooked or raw veggies, or over our Emerald-Green Garlic Sauté (page 183).

1. Place all the ingredients in the food processor or blender and blend until smooth. Alternatively, you can whisk the ingredients together in a small bowl or jar.
2. Keep this in an airtight container in the fridge for up to 5 days.

———————

1 small garlic clove

¼ cup extra-virgin olive oil

¼ cup fresh lemon juice

3 Tbsp raw sunflower seeds

1½ tsp Dijon or whole-grain mustard

1 tsp capers

¼ tsp sea salt

Pepper to taste

3–4 Tbsp water, to thin

Sunflower Seed "Caesar" Dressing

Caesar dressing is arguably one of the most popular salad dressings. But most people aren't whisking together raw eggs and anchovies themselves; no, they're buying a bottle of ready-made dressing that is loaded with unhealthy oils, additives, and sugars from the grocery store. Well, our recipe is so simple, there's no excuse not to make your own fresh, zesty dressing at home, especially when it takes less than five minutes. We're skipping the raw eggs, but the dressing still has the perfect balance of acidity and creaminess. It lasts in the fridge for up to five days, so you may even want to make a double batch.

1. Blend all the ingredients except the water in the food processor until creamy and smooth.
2. If you want the dressing a little thinner, gradually add water until the dressing reaches the consistency you like.
3. Keep it in an airtight container in the fridge for up to 5 days.

6 Tbsp toasted sesame oil

2 Tbsp tamari or coconut aminos

1 tsp grated peeled ginger root

4 tsp pure maple syrup (optional)

NUTRITION NOTE Fresh ginger root is one of the best remedies that we suggest for dealing with nausea. It also contains zinc, which supports the immune system. If you have mouth sores or are sensitive to acidic foods, this salad dressing is for you.

Low-Acidity Gingerade Dressing

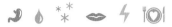

The basic template for making a salad dressing always includes some type of acid, whether from vinegar or citrus fruit, but we learned from working with our clients that sometimes acidic foods are just too irritating when you're in treatment. And yet we all know that eating bland veggies is the worst. So we've created an acid-free dressing that's full of flavor, even without the acid component. It's the perfect balance of sweet and salty, with an extra bite from the ginger.

1. Whisk all the ingredients together in a small bowl or mix together in a food processor until creamy.
2. Keep it in an airtight container in the fridge for up to a week.

Sesame oil is a great source of healthy fat and contains compounds called sesamol and sesamin that act as natural preservatives to keep the oil from turning rancid. Sesame oil also contains small amounts of omega-3 fatty acids.

6 Tbsp extra-virgin olive oil

3 Tbsp fresh lemon juice

3 tsp miso

3 tsp Dijon or whole-grain mustard

1 tsp pure maple syrup

Miso Dijon Dressing

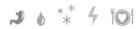

One of our good friends, who's also a nutritionist, makes the most amazing salad dressing—the type of dressing that makes you want to eat salad everyday. This recipe was inspired by that dressing. We love the combination of miso and mustard—it's salty, tangy, and slightly sweet, which makes this a good recipe to try out if your sense of taste or smell has changed.

1. Whisk all the ingredients together in a small bowl or mix in a food processor until creamy.
2. Keep it in an airtight container in the fridge for up to 5 days.

———————

1 small garlic clove, minced

5 Tbsp flax oil

3 Tbsp fresh lemon juice

2 Tbsp extra-virgin olive oil

1 Tbsp apple cider vinegar

1 tsp pure maple syrup

½ tsp Dijon mustard

Pinch of sea salt

Flax Oil Anti-Inflammation Dressing

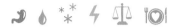

If you're in a rush, exhausted, or just want to get dinner on the table, whip up this foolproof dressing. This is version 2.0: it's enhanced with flax oil, which lends a sweeter, almost buttery taste. It couldn't be any easier to sneak some omega-3s into your diet. We like to use this dressing in Over the Rainbow Slaw (page 188).

1. Whisk all the ingredients together in a small bowl, or blend them together in a food processor.
2. Keep the dressing in an airtight container in the fridge for up to 5 days.

Studies show that omega-3 fatty acids may have a direct effect in preventing cancer by interfering with cancer cell growth and may sensitize tumors to cancer drugs, making them more effective. Flax oil is sensitive to heat and light, so it should always be stored in the refrigerator and never heated.

---

1 small garlic clove, minced

¼ cup tahini

3 Tbsp extra-virgin olive oil

2 Tbsp fresh lemon juice

¼ tsp sea salt

Water for thinning, if needed

Tahini Lemon Zest Dressing

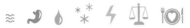

Tahini, also known as sesame butter, is my absolute favorite condiment—I drizzle it over toast, vegetables, and salads; I bake it into cookies; and sometimes I even swirl it with cacao powder for a treat. Although tahini is endlessly versatile, it's most classically paired up with lemon and garlic for a timeless Middle Eastern dressing. To buy your tahini, go to the international aisle in your grocery store; that's where you'll find the authentic stuff. This dressing can spruce up your salad, grain bowl, or any cooked vegetable dish—we find it's best when drizzled over Quinoa Tabouli (page 185). **TG**

1. Whisk all the ingredients except the water together until blended.
2. If the dressing is too thick, you can add a few spoonfuls of water until the mixture reaches your desired consistency.
3. Keep it in an airtight container in the fridge for up to 5 days.

───────────

2 cloves garlic, coarsely
   chopped

1 cup red cherry tomatoes,
   halved

1 cup yellow cherry tomatoes,
   halved

¼ cup diced red onion

1 Tbsp extra-virgin olive oil

¼ tsp sea salt

Pinch of pepper

3 Tbsp chopped fresh cilantro

2 Tbsp fresh lime juice

NUTRITION NOTE

Cooking red tomatoes increases
the amount of lycopene, a
phytonutrient that fights free
radical damage and has been
studied for its preventative
effects with prostate, lung,
and stomach cancer.

Rustic Salsa

Fresh meets rustic in our roasted version of salsa. The onions,
garlic, and tomatoes are cooked, rather than left raw, which
deepens their sweetness and makes the tomatoes literally burst
with flavor. Cooking the salsa also alleviates the irritation of raw
garlic and onion and mellows the acidity of tomatoes, which is
important if you're experiencing mouth sores or taste bud
changes. We use this in Rustic Salsa Trout (page 145), but you
can also eat it with crackers or crudités, or on chicken and
roasted vegetables.

1. Preheat the oven to 375°F and line a baking sheet with
   parchment paper.
2. Spread the garlic, red and yellow cherry tomatoes, and
   onions onto the baking sheet. Toss with the olive oil, salt,
   and pepper.
3. Roast in the oven for 20–25 minutes, or until the tomatoes
   are soft and the onions are lightly browned. After 10 minutes, give the baking sheet a quick shake to roll the tomatoes
   around.
4. Remove from the oven and let cool for 15 minutes.
5. Once cool, place the tomato mixture, cilantro, and lime
   juice in a food processor, and pulse to mix. If you like a
   rustic, chunkier look, you can omit blending it and leave it
   as is. Add more sea salt to taste.
6. Keep the salsa in an airtight jar in the fridge for up to 5 days.

If you can't find yellow cherry tomatoes, you can just use red ones. If you
don't like cilantro, you can use fresh basil instead.

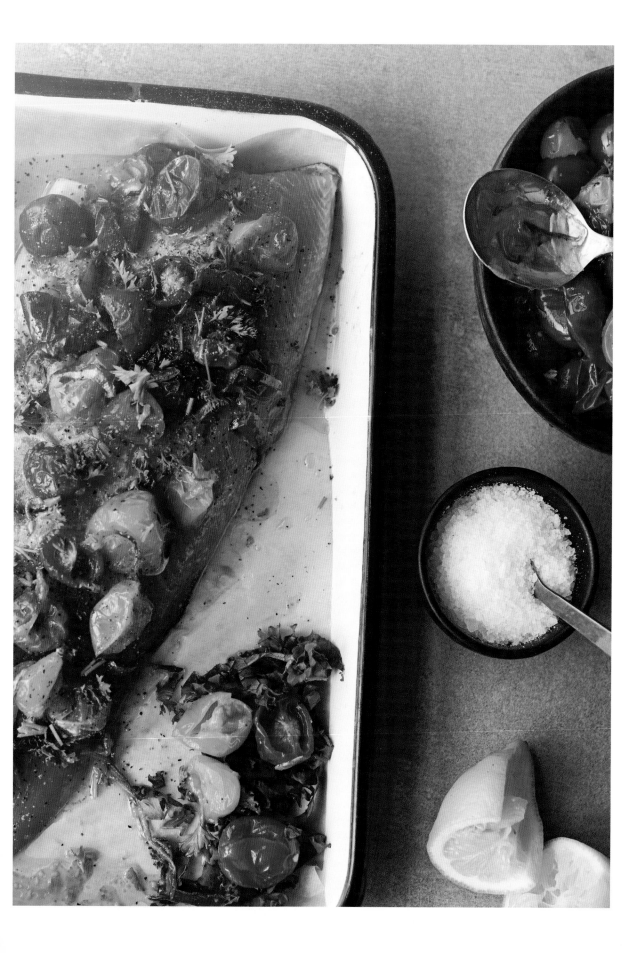

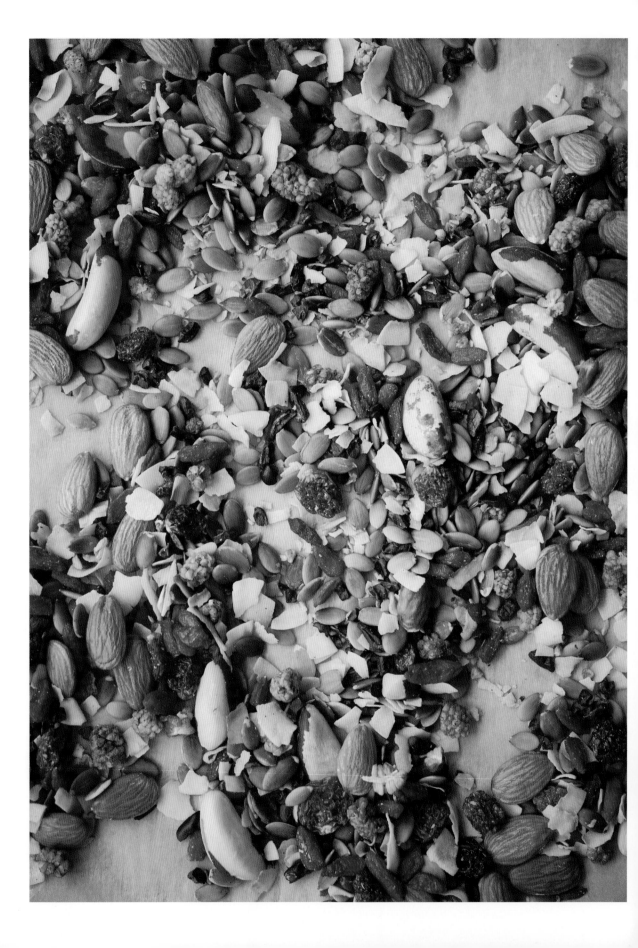

Notes

CHAPTER ONE: Facing a Diagnosis

Paccagnella A, Morello M, et al. Early nutritional intervention improves treatment tolerance and outcomes in head and neck cancer patients undergoing concurrent chemoradiotherapy. *Support Care Cancer*, vol. 18, no. 7, July 2010: pp. 837-45

Hardy, Tabitha M and Tollefsbol, Trygve O. Epigenetic diet: impact on the epigenome and cancer. *Epigenomics*, vol. 3, no. 4, August 1, 2011: pp. 503–518

CHAPTER TWO: "Let Food Be Thy Medicine"

Erasmus, Edu, *Fats that Heal, Fats the Kill*. Alive Books: 1993.

Clader, Philip C. "Functional Roles of Fatty Acids and Their Effects on Human Health." *Journal of Parenteral & Enteral Nutrition*, vol. 39, no. 1, July 2015, pp. 18S-32S.

Merendino, Nicolò et al. "Dietary ω-3 Polyunsaturated Fatty Acid DHA: A Potential Adjuvant in the Treatment of Cancer." *BioMed Research International* 2013: 310186.

Rani, Rita, and Vinod K. Kansal. "Study on Cow Ghee versus Soybean Oil on 7, 12-Dimethylbenz(a)-Anthracene Induced Mammary Carcinogenesis & Expression of Cyclooxygenase-2 & Peroxisome Proliferators Activated Receptor- Γ in Rats." *The Indian Journal of Medical Research,* vol. 133, no. 5, 2011: pp. 497–503.

Yeluri S, et al. "Cancer's Craving for Sugar: An Opportunity for Clinical Exploitation." *Journal of Cancer Research and Clinical Oncology*, no. 135, 2009: pp. 867–877.

Ben-Shmuel S, et.al. "Metabolic Syndrome, Type 2 Diabetes, and Cancer: Epidemiology and Potential Mechanisms." *Handbook of Experimental Pharmacology,* April, 2015.

Yu, Herbert, et al. "Role of the Insulin-Like Growth Factor Family in Cancer Development and Progression." JNCI: Journal of National Cancer Institute, vol. 92, no.18, 2000: pp. 1472-1489.

Jensen, Bernard. *Dr. Jensen's Guide to Better Bowel Care*. Avery a member of Penguin Putnam Inc., New York, 1999.

Elli Luca, et al. "Diagnosis of gluten related disorders: Celiac disease, wheat allergy and non-celiac gluten sensitivity." *World Journal of Gastroenterology*, vol. 21, no. 23, 2015: pp. 7110–7119.

Haas, Elson. *Staying Healthy with Nutrition*. Celestial Arts, 2006.

Eley, Helen L., et al.. "Effect of Branched-Chain Amino Acids on Muscle Atrophy in Cancer Cachexia." *The Biochemical Journal,* vol. 407. pt. 1, 2007: pp. 113–120.

"Stumped by Oxidative Stress." *Weil*, March 17, 2009, http://www.drweil.com/drw/u/QAA400537/Stumped-by-Oxidative-Stress.html.

Hong Gyeongyeon, et al. "Survey of Policies and Guidelines on Antioxidant Use for Cancer Prevention, Treatment, and Survivorship in North American Cancer Centers: What Do Institutions Perceive as Evidence?" *Integrative Cancer Therapies*, vol. 14, no. 4, 2015: pp. 305-317.

Carlsen Monica, et al. "The total antioxidant content of more than 3100 foods, beverages, spices, herbs and supplements used worldwide." *Nutrition Journal,* vol. 9, no. 3, 2010.

The George Mateljan Foundation. "Vitamin C." *The World's Healthiest Foods*, 2017, http://www.whfoods.com/genpage.php?tname=nutrient&dbid=109.

The George Mateljan Foundation. "Vitamin E." *The World's Healthiest Foods*, 2017, http://www.whfoods.com/genpage.php?tname=nutrient&dbid=111.

The George Mateljan Foundation. "Vitamin A." *The World's Healthiest Foods*, 2017, http://www.whfoods.com/genpage.php?tname=nutrient&dbid=106

The George Mateljan Foundation. "Selenium." *The World's Healthiest Foods*, 2017, http://www.whfoods.com/genpage.php?dbid=95&tname=nutrient

Block Keith I, et al. "Impact of antioxidant supplementation on chemotherapeutic efficacy: A systematic review of evidence from randomized controlled trials." *Cancer Treatment Reviews*, 2007.

Hosseini Azar, et al. "Cancer therapy and phytochemicals: evidence from clinical trials Avicenna." *Journal of Phytomedicine*, vol. 5, no. 2, 2015: pp. 84-97.

Manach Claudine, et al. "Polyphenols: food sources and bioavailability." *American Journal of Clinical Nutrition*, vol. 79, no. 5, May 2004: pp. 727-747.

Kim Do-Hee, et al. "Chemopreventive and Therapeutic Potential of Phytochemicals Targeting Cancer Stem Cells." *Current Pharmacology Reports*, vol. 1, no. 5, October 2015: pp. 302-311.

Jerrold, Simon J. "Phytochemicals & Cancer." *Journal of Chiropractic Medicine,* vol. 1, no 3, 2002: pp. 91-96.

CHAPTER THREE: Functional & Dysfunctional Foods

Gupta Charu et al. "Phytonutrients as therapeutic agents." *Journal of Complementary Integrative Medicine*, vol. 11, no. 3, 2014: pp. 151-169.

Auborn KJ, et al. "Indole-3-carbinol is a negative regulator of estrogen." *Journal of Nutrition*, vol. 133, Jul 2003: 2470S-2475S.

Gupta Parul, et al. "Phenethyl Isothiocyanate: A comprehensive review of anti-cancer mechanisms." *Biochimica et Biophysica Acta*, vol. 1846, no. 2, Dec 2014 Dec: pp. 405–424.

Auborn KJ, et al. "Indole-3-carbinol is a negative regulator of estrogen." *Journal of Nutrition*, vol. 133, Jul 2003: 2470S-2475S.

Patel Seema, et al. "Recent developments in mushrooms as anti-cancer therapeutics: a review." *3 Biotech*. vol. 2, no. 1, Mar 2012: pp. 1-15.

Fisher M, et al. "anti-cancer effects and mechanisms of polysaccharide-K (PSK): implications of cancer immunotherapy." *Anti-cancer Research*, vol. 22, no. 3, 2002: pp. 1737-1754.

Lemieszek M, et al. "Anti-cancer properties of polysaccharides isolated from fungi of the Basidiomycetes class." *Contemporary Oncology*, vol. 16, no. 4, 2012: pp. 285-289.

Kewitz Stefanie, et al. "Curcuma Contra Cancer? Curcumin and Hodgkin's Lymphoma." *Cancer Growth and Metastsis,* vol. 6, 2013: pp. 35-52.

Sa, Gaurisankar, et al. "Anti cancer effects of curcumin: cycle of life and death." *Cell Division*, vol. 3, 2008: p. 14.

Vighi, G et al. "Allergy and the Gastrointestinal System." *Clinical and Experimental Immunology,* vol. 153., suppl 1, 2008: pp. 3–6.

Yu, Ai-Qun, et al. "The potential role of probiotics in cancer prevention and treatment." *Nutrition and Cancer*, vol. 68, no. 4, May-June 2016: pp. 535-544.

Maleki, Davood, et al, "Probiotics in Cancer Prevention, Updating Evidence," *Probiotics, Prebiotics and Synbiotics: Bioactive Foods in Health Promotion,* 2016: pp. 781-791.

Nabavi, S.F. et al. "Omega 3 polyunsaturated fatty acids and cancer: lessons learned from clinical trials." *Cancer Metastasis Reviews,* vol. 34, 2015: p. 359.

Camargo, Cde Q, et al. "Fish oil supplementation during chemotherapy increases posterior time to tumor progression in colorectal cancer." *Nutrition Cancer*, vol. 68, 2016: p. 70.

Nicastro, Holly L., et al. "Garlic and onions: Their cancer prevention properties." *Cancer Prevention Research,* vol. 8, no. 3, Mar 2015: pp. 181–189.

Pandrangi A. "Cancer Chemoprevention by Garlic - A Review." *Hereditary Genetics: Current Research*, vol. 4, 2015: p. 147.

Wang, WW, et al. "Amino Acids and Gut Function." *Amino Acids*, vol. 37, no. 1, 2009 May: pp. 105-110.

Mikalauskas Saulius, et al. "Dietary glycine protects from chemotherapy-induced hepatotoxicity." *Amino Acids*, vol. 40, no. 4, 2011 April: pp. 1139-1150.

Beliveau, Richard and Denis Gingras. *Foods That Fight Cancer.* McClelland & Stewart, 2005.

Allred, C.D., et al., "Soy diets containing varying amounts of genistein stimulate growth of estrogen-dependent (MCF-7) tumors in a dose-dependent manner." *Cancer Research*, vol. 61, no. 13, 2001: p. 5045-50.

D'Adamo, CR, et. al. "Soy foods and supplementation: a review of commonly perceived health benefits and risks." *Alternative Therapies in Health and Medicine*, vol. 20, suppl 20, 2014 Winter: pp. 39-51.

Zhujun, Wang, et. al. "Inhibitory effects of small molecular peptides from Spirulina (Arthrospira) platensis on cancer cell growth." *Food & Function,* vol. 7, 2016: 781-788.

Gorjzdadeh, Homan, et. al. "Fatty acid composition of Spirulina sp., Chlorella sp. and Chaetoceros sp. microalgae and introduction as potential new sources to extinct omega 3 and omega 6." *Iranian South Medical Journal*, vol. 19, no. 2: pp. 212-224.

Noguchi, Naoto, et. al. "The Influence of *Chlorella* and Its Hot Water Extract Supplementation on Quality of Life in Patients with Breast Cancer." *Evidence-based Complementary and Alternative Medicine*, vol. 2014, 2014 March.

Yusof, Yasmin Anum Mohd, et al. "Hot Water Extract of *Chlorella Vulgaris* Induced DNA Damage and Apoptosis." *Clinics*, vol. 65, no.12, 2010: pp. 1371–1377.

Xu, XF, et. al. "Effects of sodium ferrous chlorophyll treatment on anemia of hemodialysis patients and relevant biochemical parameters." *Journal of Biological Regulators and Homeostatic Agents*, vol. 30, no. 1, 2016 Jan-Mar: pp. 135-40.

Padalia, Swati, et. al. "Multitude potential of wheatgrass juice (Green Blood): An overview." *Chronicles of Young Scientists*, vol. 1, 2010: pp. 23-8.

Liu, Haizhou, et. al. "Clove Extract Inhibits Tumor Growth and Promotes Cell Cycle Arrest and Apoptosis." *Oncology Research*, vol. 21, no.5, 2014: pp. 247–259.

Gagandeep, Dhanalakshmi, et al. "Chemopreventive effects of Cuminum cyminum in chemically induced forestomach and uterine cervix tumors in murine model systems." *Nutrition and Cancer*, vol. 47, no. 2, 2003: pp. 171-80.

Farrukh, Aqil, et. al. "Cumin extract prevents estrogen-associated breast cancer in ACI rats." *Proceedings of the 106th Annual Meeting of the American Association for Cancer Research*, 2015 Apr: pp.18-22.

Kwon, Ho-Keun et al. "Cinnamon Extract Induces Tumor Cell Death through Inhibition of NFκB and AP1." *BMC Cancer*, vol. 10, 2010: p. 392.

Panahi Y, Saadat A, Sahebkar A, et al. "Effect of ginger on acute and delayed chemotherapy-induced nausea and vomiting: a pilot, randomized, open-label clinical trial." *Integrative Cancer Therapies,* vol. 11, no. 3, 2012, pp. 204-11.

Park, Gwang Hun et al. "Anti-Cancer Activity of Ginger (*Zingiber Officinale*) Leaf through the Expression of Activating Transcription Factor 3 in Human Colorectal Cancer Cells." *BMC Complementary and Alternative Medicine,* vol. 14, 2014, p. 408.

Akimoto, Miho et al. "anti-cancer Effect of Ginger Extract against Pancreatic Cancer Cells Mainly through Reactive Oxygen Species-Mediated Autotic Cell Death." *PLOS ONE,* vol. 10, no. 5, 2015.

Hamidpour, Rafie et al. "Cinnamon from the Selection of Traditional Applications to Its Novel Effects on the Inhibition of Angiogenesis in Cancer Cells and Prevention of Alzheimer's Disease, and a Series of Functions such as Antioxidant, Anticholesterol, Antidiabetes, Antibacterial, Antifungal, Nematicidal, Acaracidal, and Repellent Activities." *Journal of Traditional and Complementary Medicine*, vol. 5, no. 2, 2015: pp. 66–70.

Tang, E. L., et. al. "*Petroselinum crispum* has antioxidant properties, protects against DNA damage and inhibits proliferation and migration of cancer cells." Journal of the Science of Food and Agriculture, vol. 95, 2015: pp. 2763–2771.

Borrás-Linares, I., et. al. "A bioguided identification of the active compounds that contribute to the antiproliferative/cytotoxic effects of rosemary extract on colon cancer cells." *Food Chemical Toxicology*, vol. 80, 2015 Jun: pp. 215-22.

Fitsiou E, et. al. "Phytochemical Profile and Evaluation of the Biological Activities of Essential Oils Derived from the Greek Aromatic Plant Species *Ocimum basilicum, Mentha spicata, Pimpinella anisum* and *Fortunella margarita*." *Molecules,* vol. 21, no. 8, 2016: p. 1069.

Larsson, Susanna C., et. al. "Meat Consumption and Risk of Colorectal Cancer: A Meta-Analysis of Prospective Studies." *International Journal of Cancer,* vol. 119, no. 11, December 2006: pp. 2657-2664.

Lippi, Giuseppe, et. al. "Meat consumption and cancer risk: a critical review of published meta-analyses." *Critical Reviews in Oncology/Hematology*, vol. 97, 2016 January: pp. 1-14.

Cross, Amanda J., et. al. "Impact of Food Preservation, Processing, and Cooking on Cancer Risk." *Carcinogenic and Anticarcinogenic Food Components*, 2005: pp. 97-105.

Hicks, Cherrill. "Give up dairy products to beat cancer." *The Telegraph*, 2 June 2014. http://www.telegraph.co.uk/foodanddrink/healthyeating/10868428/Give-up-dairy-products-to-beat-cancer.html

Crowe, Francesca L., et. al. "The Association between Diet and Serum Concentrations of IGF-I, IGFBP-1, IGFBP-2, and IGFBP-3 in the European Prospective Investigation into Cancer and Nutrition." *Cancer Epidemiology, Biomarkers & Prevention*, vol. 18, no. 5, May 2009.

Yu, Herbert, et. al. "Role of the Insulin-Like Growth Factor Family in Cancer Development and Progression." *Journal of National Cancer Institute*, vol. 92, no. 18, 2000: pp. 1472-1489.

Jianqin, Sun, et. al. "Effects of milk containing only A2 beta casein versus milk containing both A1 and A2 beta casein proteins on gastrointestinal physiology, symptoms of discomfort, and cognitive behavior of people with self-reported intolerance to traditional cows' milk." *Nutrition Journal*, vol. 15, 2015.

Hu J, Vecchia C. La, et. al. "Glycemic Index, Glycemic Load and Cancer Risk." Annals of Oncology, vol. 24, no. 1, 2013: pp. 245-251.

Mullie P, Koechlin A, et. al. "Relation between Breast Cancer and High Glycemic Index or Glycemic Load: A Meta-analysis of Prospective Cohort Studies." *Critical Reviews in Food Science and Nutrition*, vol. 56, no. 1, 2016: pp. 152-9.

Fuchs Michael A., Sato Kaori, et al. "Sugar-Sweetened Beverage Intake and Cancer Recurrence and Survival in CALGB 89803 (Alliance)." *PLoS One*, vol. 9, no. 6, 2014 Jun.

Orgel, Etan, et. al. "The Links Between Insulin Resistance, Diabetes, and Cancer." *Current Diabetes Reports*, vol. 13, no. 2, 2013 April: pp. 213–222.

Arcidiacono, Biagio, et. al. "Insulin Resistance and Cancer Risk: An Overview of the Pathogenetic Mechanisms." *Experimental Diabetes Research*, vol. 2012, 2012 April.

Brown, Kirsty, et al. "Diet-Induced Dysbiosis of the Intestinal Microbiota and the Effects on Immunity and Disease." *Nutrients*, vol. 4, no. 8, 2012 Aug: pp. 1095–1119.

Sanchez Albert, et al. "Role of sugars in human neutrophilic phagocytosis." *American Journal* of Clinical Nutrition, vol. 26 no. 11, November 1973: pp. 1180-1184.

Strawbridge, Holly. "Artificial sweeteners: sugar-free, but at what cost?" *Harvard Health Publications*, updated 2015 December 8. http://www.health.harvard.edu/blog/artificial-sweeteners-sugar-free-but-at-what-cost-201207165030.

Soffritti, Morando, et. al. "The Carcinogenic Effects of Aspartame: The Urgent Need for Regulatory Re-Evaluation." *American Journal of Industrial Medicine*, vol. 57, no. 4, 2014: pp. 383–397.

Praud Delphine, Rota Matteo, et. al. "Cancer incidence and mortality attributable to alcohol consumption." *International Journal of Cancer*, vol. 138, no. 6, March 2016: pp. 1380-1387.

CHAPTER FOUR: Eating to Combat Common Side Effects

Haas, Elson. *Staying Healthy with Nutrition*. Celestial Arts, 2006.

CHAPTER FIVE: Preparing the Kitchen

Dich J, Zahm SH, et al. "Pesticides and cancer." *Cancer Causes Control*. vol. 8, no. 3, May 1997, pp. 420-43.

Krol, Walter J. "Removal of Trace Pesticide Residues from Produce." The Connecticut Agricultural Experiment Station, 2012, www.ct.gov/caes/cwp/view.asp?a=2815&q=376676.

Bolton, Jason and Bushway, Alfred, et. al. "Best Ways to Wash Fruits and Vegetables." University of Maine Department of Food Science and Human Nutrition, and Cooperative Extension, 2013, https://extension.umaine.edu/publications/4336e/.

Chauhan R, Kumari B, et. al. "Effect of fruit and vegetable processing on reduction of synthetic pyrethroid residues." Reviews Environmental Contamination and Toxicology, vol. 229, December 2013, pp. 89-110.

Abels, Caroline. Pasture-raised vs. grass-fed: What's the difference? Humaneitarian. 28 September 2013. Web. 15 July 2016.

Ley, Sylvia H et al. "Associations between Red Meat Intake and Biomarkers of Inflammation and Glucose Metabolism in Women." *The American Journal of Clinical Nutrition,* vol. 99, no. 2, February 2014, pp. 352–360.

Environmental Working Group. "EWG's Healthy Home Tips: Tip 6 - Skip the Non-Stick to Avoid the Dangers of Teflon." *Environmental Working Group*, 2017, http://www.ewg.org/research/healthy-home-tips/tip-6-skip-non-stick-avoid-dangers-teflon.

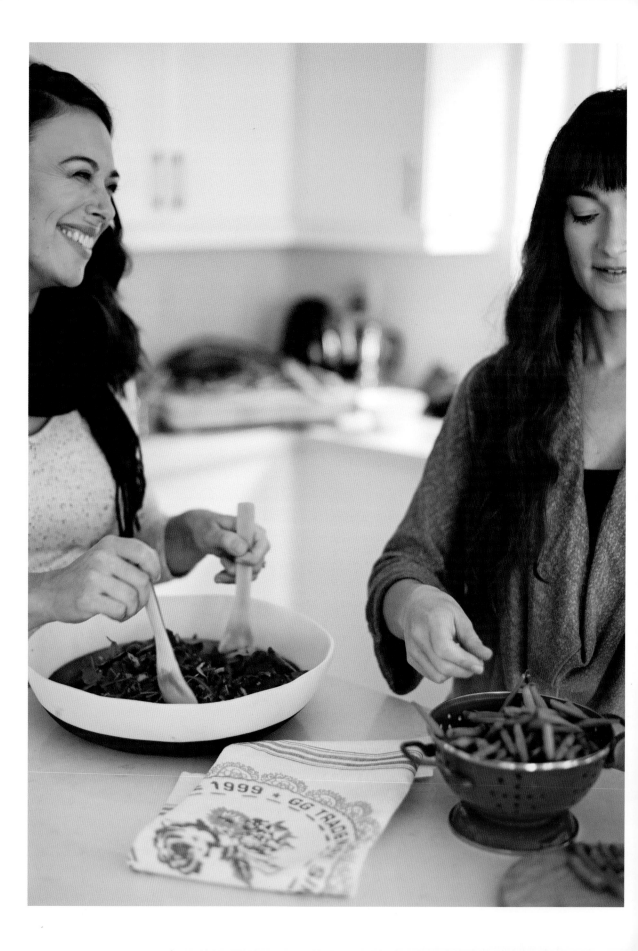

Acknowledgements

FROM SG AND TG:

To our dear clients, readers, followers, and subscribers: We thank you for your ongoing support, encouragement and belief in us. We have written this book because of you.

To our wonderful team at Appetite by Random House: Bhavna Chauhan—we are so honored to have you as our editor and grateful for all of the countless hours you put into this book, always guiding and supporting us. Thank you to Robert McCullough for seeing the potential in this book. Kelly Hill, thank you for your beautiful design vision. Thanks also to the entire editorial team for *your* keen attention to detail.

Daniel Alexander: Without you, this book would not have been possible. Thank you so much for putting your everything into creating these beautiful photographs and for always encouraging us to be better.

To our photography support team: A huge thank you to both Michelle Margulis and Amanda Reid for your incredible, talented make up skills and for making our hair beautiful. Jenn and Dave Stark—thank you for your help with capturing candid, natural photos. Thank you Mia Shulman and Benji Guth for letting us take over your kitchen more than once. Maggie Walker, thank you for always helping us out on set and making things run smoothly.

Suzanne Brandreth and Paige Sisley: Thank you for making this book come to life and for your belief in us. And, to the rest of the team at CookeMcDermid—thank you for your continued support.

To our incredible recipe testers, Rebecca Moutoussidis, Samantha Era, Jess Tilley, Sandy Seliga, and Carley Nadine: Your insight and careful preparation of so many recipes made this book possible.

To Jaye McKenzie: thank you for being our teacher, cheerleader and positivity coach. You were there when this journey began and we can't thank you enough for all that you have taught us.

To our friends and family who constantly asked how the book was going, and who were so invested to see it come to life: thank you. And, thank you to the ones who told us they would be first in line to buy their copy when the book comes out!

FROM SG:

Daniel, you make my world better every day and I am so grateful for your wisdom, laughter and love. Thank you for always believing in me, cleaning up the kitchen at the end of the day, and for being my partner through it all.

To my family: my parents—thank you for supporting everything I've ever wanted to do and for your unwavering encouragement, especially on this book. Your love of good, nourishing food made everything I do possible. And to Leda, thank you always for being there and for making the best sourdough bread I've ever had.

Lastly, thank you to Ann, for being the inspiration that kept me writing this book.

FROM TG:

To Bram: Thank you for being YOU. You are my voice of reason, my source of peace, calm, groundedness, and love. Your unwavering belief in me astounds me and keeps me going. The making of this book has been a long, long process that certainly could not have happened without you.

To Jackson: To think that this book was written in your first year of life still amazes me. You are truly the greatest thing that has ever happened to me. Thank you for being the best source of toddler comic relief and for being the greatest teacher I have ever had. And to Baby Boo Boo, you're still swimming in my belly as I write this and your brother lovingly has given you this name. You've come along for the ride on this journey and I wouldn't have it any other way.

To my parents, Lisa and Barry: Jillian and I are always in disbelief about how lucky we are to have you as our parents. You do *so much* for us and your level of unconditional support and love is beyond conception.

To Jillian: Your innate, kind, loving spirit is an inspiration to me and everyone that surrounds you. Thank you for being willing to literally drop anything and everything at a moment's notice just to help me.

Symptoms and Recipes Index

Index